TORRENTIAL MIST

Sean Bellamy Rice Sr.

ISBN 978-1-64468-491-7 (Paperback)
ISBN 978-1-64468-492-4 (Digital)

Covenant Books, Inc.
11661 Hwy 707
Murrells Inlet, SC 29576
www.covenantbooks.com

In "Torrential Mist," Sean Bellamy Rice, Sr. gives voice to painful diseases that many people around the world have experienced and are experiencing right now. Sean's life and his painful memories about his extreme situation and how he dealt with them, I think will help anyone who finds themselves in traumatic situations. The book covers his life from the time he was twelve years old all the way until the present. As his big brother I have known him all of his life and I am in awe of his positiveness in the face of all his pain and disease. Even though he is younger than me, I have to say that he is my hero. The book is so compelling and interesting, I could not put it down. Although I haven't gone through what he has experienced, it even encouraged me, with my small problems. I believe anyone who is going through trauma, disease, pain or even mental anguish will be helped and encouraged, with God, to live a happy and triumphant life by reading "Torrential Mist."

Edgar L. Rice, IV

CONTENTS

LUCAS DRIVE

Growing up in Fort Worth, Texas, as an African American in the mid-1960s was like any other all-American town. We listened to the sounds of Motown and living in Fort Worth, Texas, we also loved the Dallas Cowboys. I was born in 1963—the year President Kennedy was assassinated. I was the youngest child of Edgar and Exeree Rice's eight children—four boys and four girls, where some were so age separated we hardly knew each other. I don't remember my oldest brother and sister ever living with us because my earliest recollection of them was during their college years. Shelia was at North Texas State (now known as the University of North Texas), and Joc was at Prairie View.

My first address was twenty-five-oh-five Lucas Drive. The way we would say it had a distinct rhythm, like poetry rolling off the tongue "Twenty-five-oh-five Lucas Drive." All eight of us Rice children lived in that house at one time or another. We all started school at Rosedale Park Elementary School. Rosedale Park was right around the corner from our house, and we all walked to school. There was a principle at Rosedale Park, whose name was Mrs. Walton. She ran the school like a dictatorship. She didn't spare the rod, if you know what I mean. She believed in discipline. Each of the eight children in our household had a relationship with Mrs. Walton, and unlike most public-school administrators now, she had a relationship with us children and our parents.

Most of the kids in our family went to the sixth grade before leaving Rosedale Park to go to Dunbar Middle School. In the late sixties and early seventies, our government started a new integration program. I was probably in the second grade, while my sister Carlotta was in the third grade. We were both bussed to a school in a predominately white neighborhood called East Handley Elementary School. It was somewhat of a culture shock in the beginning, since we had never gone to school with white kids, but maybe, I was just too young and naive to know what was really going on around me, but I didn't notice any racial conflict.

I was a student at East Handley till I was in the fourth grade when my parents decided to move to a small town in east Texas, called Jefferson. The only real claim to fame Jefferson has is its place in history. It is the fifth oldest city in Texas. All our grandparents lived in Jefferson, and I remember visiting all the time as a child. My father's mother had passed away a few years before we moved, and his father, my grandfather, was living all alone. My parents wanted to move there to take care of my grandfather. There were only four children left at home during this move—two boys and two girls. My brother and I were virtually indifferent about the move, but my sisters saw it as a social disaster living in "the country."

Daddy, what his children called him was the youngest of two children in his immediate family. He was also the third of six generations to carry the name Edgar. He was known in our small town as Brother, and his sister Verna was known as Sister. All their nieces and nephews would address them as Uncle Brother and Aunt Sister, which could be confusing to people outside of our circle. Normally, you will hear the title Brother in church, but that wasn't the case with Daddy. I never saw him inside a church, except at MawMaw's and PawPaw's, his mother and father's, funerals and my mother's funeral. He would always say, "My Mama would have me in church almost on a daily basis during my adolescence, and that was enough church for me."

Daddy had other names around town such as the Bar-B-Q Man or the Watermelon Man. My father was a hardworking man who always seemed to have at least two jobs and a hustle on the side; hence, all the names he was known by around town. He was also known as the man you could get ten or twenty bucks from, if you were a bit short on funds. He would loan you a few bucks at some exorbitant interest rate, but it was a valuable service for many African

Americans in our community. Working was very important to him, in an attempt to provide for such a large family.

My mother, Exeree, was one of fourteen children in her family, of which there were three girls and eleven boys. They were all very fair skinned. Many of the fourteen children had the resemblance of our Native American population. It's ironic. Despite all the children's fair skin, my grandfather, Grover Cleveland Jefferson, had an extremely dark complexion. Mama especially had the high cheek bones you would associate with Native Americans.

Mama was a homemaker/beautician, who had many other vocation beside her occupations. She always found time to be a part of my siblings' lives and mine. She was available for every situation that came up with her children. In Jefferson, our town, all social events took place in the city limits, but we lived about six miles from the town in more of a rural area. With our old worn-out cars, and not much discretionary income, Mama was determined to get us to town for any event, club, or team we wanted to be a part of.

In the big scheme of things, my family would have been considered lower middle class in the socioeconomic spectrum, but as a young child, I was so protected by my parents and elder siblings I didn't understand the struggles of raising a family in this environment.

The dynamic between my brothers and sisters was evenly spaced to where there was always a boy and a girl together. My sister Shelia is the oldest, but my brother Edgar IV (Joc) carries himself as the eldest of the two. My sister Gala is the next in line and the one who took on most of my father's character. I suppose most African American families had a black power sign wielding, outspoken, militant during the late sixties and early seventies, and my brother Malcolm represented this persona for our family. After Malcolm, the mold was broken from girl, boy, girl, boy, to another boy. Cedric is the next sibling to come along. Cedric is very stoic in his demeanor, but he looks like my mother's mother, Millie Jefferson, who was anything but stoic. In fact, she was quite the little general in the way she carried herself. She was small in stature and extremely bow-legged. She was also very fair skinned. She could almost pass as a white woman.

My parents got back on track with another girl named Jill, who was next in the family tree. Jill's first name is Iva, and I didn't know this until I was about eight years old, when I heard a friend of hers call her Iva Jill. She had a bubbly self-confidence I've always admired. Jill is an intellectual who would always correct our grammar. Next is my sister Carlotta, who in many ways seems like the baby of the family. Then along came me, a shy, unassuming all-American boy, growing up like millions of us, not knowing what to expect from this vast an amazing world, and not yet realizing all the tragedy and triumph I would encounter along my journey.

When I first became conscious of my name, I wondered why my parents would do such a thing to me, like naming me Sean Bellamy Rice. The last name alone was enough for the children at school to ridicule and make fun of. My first name was fine as long, as no one had to read it. When teachers would do roll call, they would immediately mispronounce it. While reading my name, they would pronounce it as "Seen." I still know people who kid me about that pronunciation. Sean is a Gaelic name that's typically found in Scotland, but in urban America in the 1960s, there weren't many Seans.

After witnessing how children treated my first and last name, I wouldn't dare tell my middle name. My mother said she got my middle name, Bellamy, from the last name of a news reporter in those days. As I grew older, I came to realize how my parents went to great efforts to give all their children names that would transcend our circumstances.

Of course, I had a couple of nicknames growing up. During my time of teething as a child, I would literally teeth on every wooden surface in our house. When I became of age, my family would show me the tables and bedpost and windowsills around the house with teeth marks. Hence the nickname Bug. As I said earlier, Sean has a Gaelic derivative and is usually found in Scotland or Ireland, so my family would call me "Sean, Sean, the Leprechaun." There was something about the sound of that nickname that I grew an immense appreciation for.

I've made it to the age of fifty-three and not without some tremendous obstacles before me. My basic mode of transportation is usually walking, since I haven't owned a car for several years. Many people in my neighborhood recognize me since they see me walking around town, but the knowledge of the struggles of my life go unnoticed to the naked eye. One thing I've noticed in my lifetime is a very cliché proposition everybody is going through something. You can start with the old adage "more money, more problems" because most of us who aren't rich feel that money can solve all our problems. Then you go from rich people problems to the starving child in a third-world country. Everyone in between these two extremes is dealing with something.

My affliction is my renal failure that causes me to be a dialysis patient. I'm also a double below-the-knee amputee. Usually, while out in public, I will wear long pants to hide my prosthesis, mostly in an effort to hide the truth. That's a hang up I'll have to deal with. When I'm in my wheelchair and not wearing my prosthesis, most adults try to ignore my disability. To be honest with you, I'm not sure how people should react. Most children look in amazement almost in a state of hypnosis. The first time I took my prosthesis off in front of my granddaughter, who was three years old at the time, she ran to my son, pointing and saying, "Look, Daddy, look!" She has since become very accustom to my amputee situation.

Living as an amputee has its limitations, but living with renal failure has much more dire consequences. Yet I spend more time thinking about the amputations. That's a reflection upon our society as we want to look good for the world to see. With renal failure, you have to constantly watch your diet and keep fluid intake extremely low. You also have to make sure you don't miss dialysis appointments. These things are essentially second nature to me, but my amputations are always on my mind.

Both of the disabilities I live with on a daily bases have caused me to reflect on the life I've lived to this point, and it sometimes makes me wonder "Why me?" and why not someone else in this world of over seven and a half billion people, an evil person perhaps, who might be more deserving. I'm basically a good person who has always been kind and respectful to my fellow man. Sometimes, I've asked myself, *Why is God punishing me in this way?* Upon my reflection, I realized Jesus addressed this issue in Mark 10:17–22 when he said "No one is good except God alone." Once I grasped this concept, I realized maybe I'm not the good person I thought I was, and it gave me the impetus to look at my life from God's perspective, rather than my own.

It made me reach to the other end of the spectrum. I started to think the sin in my life was so heinous God was paying me back for my indiscretion. I believe God takes a special interest in every individual, and he gives us all opportunity for redemption. The Bible tells us in Romans 6:23 that "the wages of sin is death but the gift of God is eternal life through Jesus Christ." The wages of sin aren't "amputation" or "renal failure," so I was able to dismiss that notion of my predicament being sin based. It came to my attention that the things we go through in life are not necessarily the wages of sin, although doing the wrong thing can have terribly extreme consequences.

A scripture that has always allowed me to view my life as a blessing from God is in John 9:11, where Jesus's disciples asked him about a blind man. They asked if his blindness was because of his own sin or the sin of his parents. Jesus explained this man wasn't blind because of sin, but he was blind so the glory of God might be displayed in his life. The only conclusion I can come up with is that God has given me an opportunity to show how he is working in my life through the disabilities I've suffered from.

PUNT, PASS, AND KICK

My earliest memories were consumed with thoughts of becoming a professional football player. From the age of five, I remember going to see my older brothers play while they were in junior high and high school. Seeing them in their uniforms gave me a sense of pride. The only thing that could surpass my sense of pride in them was if I could wear a uniform like that and become a football player myself. I never considered a plan B for my life because it was football or bust. As a child, it was never understood that statistics were very much against this career choice, so I chased this with all my heart.

The games I attended at an early age were during the day, but during the State Fair of Texas, I got an opportunity to see my oldest brother, Joc, play in the Cotton Bowl, at night, under the lights. My brother played at Prairie View A&M University, and they would always play Bishop College (today, it's called Paul Quinn College) at the state fair. This was a big deal among African Americans in the state of Texas, during the mid- to late-1960s. Of course, from my point of view, it was the most enormous spectacle I had ever seen. When most people think of historically black colleges and universities when it comes to athletics, they think of the marching bands, but for me, it was all about football. During the 1960s, the HBCU were a hotbed for African American talent, making enormous contributions in the NFL. All these larger-than-life players on the field under the lights of the Cotton Bowl were enough to solidify my ambition of becoming a football player.

After the game, my parents and my other siblings went down to where the players were coming off the field to talk with my brother. Joc was always huge in my eyes, but seeing him in his uniform made him look like a giant to a five-year-old. I was so inflated with pride for my brother I talked to everyone I could about how my brother was a football player, and someday, I would be a football player.

My family continued on with our lives at 2505 Lucas Drive in Fort Worth, Texas. Both Joc and Shelia were off to college. I can't imagine what it must have been like financially for my parents having two children in college and six children at home to feed and clothe, but they did it on a daily basis without complaint. During this time, my family was stricken with a life-altering circumstance. My mother was diagnosed with breast cancer. I didn't realize how protected I was by my parents from the slings and arrows of life a family can endure. I continued to play, go to school, and think about my future as a football player, while my parents and older siblings were saddled with this information about my mother's cancer diagnoses.

My mother was a simple woman who didn't seek to impress anyone, but her demeanor was such that everyone who was exposed to her was very impressed. When I was a small child, I was embarrassed by my mother's age. Most kids my age had much younger mothers because they didn't have siblings as old as mine. As I got older, I started to realize how fortunate I was to have a mother with the experience and strength to raise eight children. I appreciate her even more as time goes by.

When my mother was diagnosed with breast cancer, it was a time that could have destroyed most families, but because of my mother's strength, she held everything together. After I became an adult, my brother, Joc, told me that had my mother passed away from cancer—and back in those days, death was a strong possibility—my sister Carlotta and I would have lived with him and his wife, Sarah. My life would have been very different had this occurred, but I can't say if it would have been better or worse. Fortunately, my mother was a breast cancer survivor.

Growing up watching my brothers play football really made an impression upon me to where I naturally thought this was my calling in life. I always played with the neighborhood kids, and in my own eyes, I was an above-average player. One Christmas, myself and a few kids in the neighborhood got Dallas Cowboy football uniforms. They were more like glorified Halloween costumes, rather than football uniforms because the helmets and the pads couldn't survive any extreme impact, but for us kids, it didn't matter. Those uniforms made us feel like professional football players. Every day, after that Christmas, we would meet in someone's front yard to play the most important game of our lives.

The games continued for a while, but even when there wasn't a game, I would be in my front yard, in my uniform, playing an imaginary game of my own. Many of our neighbors must have thought I was quite peculiar playing football with my uniform on in the front yard all by myself, but to me, it was the beginning of my destiny.

At the age of nine, I got an opportunity to play football for the YMCA. Playing with the YMCA required an entry fee my parents couldn't afford, so I had to sale cookies to come up with the funds to pay my entry fee. Once again, this was an endeavor my sainted mother had to take on. This was my first attempt at being part of a real football team. Little did I know it was basically a bunch of kids running around in circles, and I wasn't the star I thought I would be. There were no spectacular plays or last second touchdowns where I would be the hero. This experience taught me that football is the ultimate team sport, and no one player can accomplish anything without his teammates.

We moved to Jefferson soon after my first team experience, but my dream of becoming a professional football player was never squelched. So I continued to put my uniform on and go to the front yard to play by myself. There weren't any other kids in the neighborhood to play with in Jefferson. At times, Cedric, who was playing high school football, and was very good, would go outside with me and teach me plays he knew from his experience in the game. We had a large front yard, so we could always throw long bombs and run deep pass patterns without any problems.

When I was ten years old, I heard about this competition coming up called Punt, Pass, and Kick. All the boys in my school were excited about the event. There were certain boys at my school who were preordained as the best athletes in the school and were predicted to win the competition. I was extremely shy as a child, and though I felt I could compete, my shyness didn't allow me to show my confidence among others. The concept of practice was quite foreign to me, but the concept of playing football and having fun was second nature. So every day after school, I would go to the front yard and throw the football, punt, and kick to get ready for the competition.

Finally, the day of the competition came, and I was so nervous almost to the point of not competing. The object of the competition was to accumulate the most yardage in the three phases of the competition. When I worked on these things at home, I discovered I could throw the ball well, and I could kick decently. But when I punted, the ball would go straight up into the air. Sometimes, when I punted, I would have to run to keep the ball from hitting the top of my head. I didn't really understand God's favor in these type of matters, but I was always taught that good things come to those who pray. So I prayed that God would allow me to get a good punt. Well, my punt managed to go out in front of me, and my pass and kick seemed to be pretty good as well.

After the competition, all the kids sat in the bleachers to wait for the announcement of the winners of each age category. Even though I was somewhat confident in my performance, my shyness wouldn't allow me to conceive the thought of possibly winning this competition. The announcer started with the eight- and nine-year-old winners. When he got to the ten-year-old winners, I was trembling inside. First, he announced the third-place winner for the ten-year-olds, and it wasn't me. Then, he announced the second-place winner for the ten-year-olds, and once again, it wasn't me. At this point, the anxiety started to build within my mind, but I didn't want to give the outward impression that this meant anything to me. So I sat with a calm demeanor as the announcer started to announce the winner. "And the winner of the ten-year-old 1973 Punt, Pass, and Kick Competition is…Sean Rice!" I walked down the bleachers to receive my trophy, as if it was common for me, but I was turning flips on the inside. This was my first real football accomplishment, and I thought this was just the beginning. Today, Punt, Pass, and Kick, tomorrow the NFL.

All the winners in the competition were eligible to compete in the regional tournament in Mount Pleasant, Texas, in a couple of weeks. In my mind, I would go there and win without any problems. It never occurred to me the competition would be greater, and my concept of practice wasn't to get better. So I didn't really practice at all after my first-place finish. Needless to say, I was extremely unprepared for the regional competition, and I got totally humiliated.

After the regional competition, life went on as usual. I continued to go to school every day, and every day after school, I was back in the front yard, by myself, pursuing my dream of becoming a professional football player. My brother Cedric had moved out to go to college, so I didn't have him to run plays and throw passes. But I managed to keep my imaginary games going. I was in the fifth grade by this time, and in just two more years, I would be able to play football on a real team.

I started to develop an interest in basketball because we played in PE at school. I seemed to have some ability in this sport as well as football. My friends and I would play basketball every chance we got. Sometimes, we would meet on the weekends on the courts at the high school to play. Basketball was fun, but it didn't deter me from my dream of being a football player. Others in my age group just floated with the seasons. It didn't matter to the other kids whether it was football, basketball, or baseball. I tried my hand at baseball, but for some reason, I didn't seem to get an opportunity to play. I tried to get involved in baseball, but it was very difficult for me. It didn't seem so difficult for the white kids in my school to get involved, and I am, by no means, trying to cast any aspersions on the community in which I grew up, But I think it was a sign of the times. My brothers never played baseball, so I developed the attitude that baseball was a white man's game.

When I got to the seventh grade, I wasn't thinking about who the teachers would be or what classes would be like. It was all about football, baby! I was so excited when we went to the field house to get our pads and helmets. Life was wonderful until practice started. It seemed to be lots of repetition and running that I wasn't prepared for. I was one of the smaller kids on our team, so my goal was to play wide receiver. The coaches saw I had some throwing ability, so they asked me to play quarterback, while still allowing me to play wide receiver.

Practice was extremely difficult for me during this period, but there was no way I would quit. I started to lose a lot of weight, and I attributed this to the hard practice sessions. While watching television one night, I saw a commercial about diabetes and the symptoms surrounding the disease. The commercial talked about frequent urination, extreme thirst, and weight lost. I was experiencing all these symptoms. The frequent urination was so bad I was wetting the bed constantly at night. This wasn't normal for me, and it deeply concerned my mother. Before I saw that commercial, I assumed all the symptoms I was having were due to the hard workouts I was going through in football practice.

My mother decided to take me to the doctor and have the situation checked out. I went through a series of test, and on the day of my first football game, I got the news. I have type 1, or what it was called back then, juvenile diabetes. I was told I would be admitted to the hospital that day, and I wouldn't be allowed to play football for the rest of the year. This was devastating news, and my heart was completely and utterly broken. My dream, for as long as I could remember, was over. When I was finally admitted to the hospital, I sat in my room and cried my eyes out. I really had no idea what diabetes was and what type of impact it would have on the rest of my life.

I spent the next two weeks in the hospital, although it felt more like an eternity, learning about drastic diet changes and taking insulin. Diabetes is a disease that develops when the pancreas stops secreting insulin. In my case, as of most with juvenile diabetes, I had to start this regimen of injections once a day for the rest of my life. The nurses in the hospital gave me instruction on how to inject the medication, as well as showing me the different locations on my body where I could inject. I always thought the easiest injection site would be my arm, in my triceps. Other locations were the front of my upper thigh, the side of my stomach, and my buttocks.

Before they allowed me to inject myself, I had to practice. They gave me a syringe with saline in it with an orange. They told me the best way to simulate injecting my skin would be to inject the orange. To me, this wasn't a very good simulation because I felt the skin of the orange was much tougher than mine. No matter how much I practiced with the orange, I never could simulate the sting of injecting my own body. My mother also learned how to inject the insulin as well. I had to move the injection sight to different locations, and I couldn't reach my buttocks, so my mother did the honors whenever I had to inject there.

While in the hospital, I would lie in bed at night and wonder what would become of me with this disease I was so unfamiliar with and is already taking me through a whirlwind of changes I would have never imagined for myself. It was more than my twelve-year-old mind could process. I wasn't aware of how common the disease was. I just felt I was all alone in this black hole. Church wasn't a priority focus in my life. In fact, I seldom went to church, but God was discussed in my home. And I felt a certain spirituality within me. Through all this, I developed a sense that this was God's plan for my life and that he would make this disease work out to my advantage. This is how my juvenile thought process allowed me to deal with the circumstances facing me.

I remember my classmates writing me letters of encouragement while in the hospital. Most of the girls talked about how they missed me in class or hoping I would get well soon. The boys, however, told me about our first football game in their letters. Needless to say, I was very excited to read the boys' letters talking about certain plays from the game and who scored touchdowns. Those letters helped me to visualize the game, but I was still heartbroken over the fact that I wasn't able to compete.

After learning the basics about diabetes and how to take care of myself, I was released from the hospital. My life seemed a bit fragile after the diagnosis. I wasn't sure what I could do without causing major damage to my body. Could I run? The biggest change was my diet. My mother was strict on how she cooked food for me and what she fed me. Her influence in my diet went a long way in contributing to my health. By this time, the only children at home were Jill, Carlotta, and me. With all the attention surrounding me with diabetes, I can't help but wonder if Jill and Carlotta felt neglected in some way. They probably didn't feel neglected. My mother had a way of making everyone feel love and respect.

I finally went back to school, and that took some getting used to. No one at my school brought their lunch. Most black kids ate in the cafeteria, while most white kids, who were considered more affluent, would buy chips, soda, and other things like that from the vending machines at the school. My mother would give me food for lunch, based on her knowledge of what a diabetic should eat. I was very insecure about carrying lunch every day when no one else was doing this.

There was another child in my seventh-grade class, Jonny Ray, who had been diagnosed with diabetes, although his was diagnosed a couple of years earlier than mine. I tried to draw on his experience in handling the disease, but I noticed how he lived more of a normal life than what I felt my life had become. My parents, mostly my mother, was very protective, and she decided specific lunch would be best for me. She also made me carry hard candy in case of an insulin reaction. I never saw Jonny taking these kinds of precautions with the disease. He functioned well with our peers, and he seemed quite happy. For the next few years, Johnny and I would often discuss our issues as diabetics, but I would always look to Johnny as the expert on the subject since he had more experience, and he seemed so comfortable with this.

So I continued my education in the seventh grade, but I was extremely upset that I couldn't play football. I was allowed to continue to be a part of the team by becoming a manager. It sounds impressive, but to me, I was just a glorified water boy. This was a long way from being the stand-out athlete I envisioned for my life, but at least, I was still a part of the team.

We ended up playing for the district title against Mount Pleasant that year. In many ways, Mount Pleasant was superior to our team, but we competed for four quarters. And they eventually beat us 14 to 8. It was the end of the football season, and we were very optimistic about the next year's team.

As football season ended, basketball season began. Basketball was much different from football in that we had tryouts for the team, and only fifteen individuals could be part of the team. With football, anyone who wanted to be part of the team could participate. My doctor did allow me to try out for the team, so this made me quite happy.

Once tryouts started, it was evident who the great players would be. It was also evident who would make the team because of reputation of being a good athlete. I wasn't either the greatest athlete or a great player, but I was a good player and a decent athlete. I was known as one who worked hard despite the disease I was diagnosed with during the football season. The attributes I did possess gave me some influence with the coach as he chose his players.

There were two cuts before our coach chose the final team. Even though I felt good about my chances of getting past the first cut, there was still much anxiety while waiting for coach to put up the first list on the field house door. As I walked up to look at the list, I prayed within because this was the most important thing in the world to me at the time. I started reading the names from the top, and as I past each name, my heart sank a bit lower until I saw my name on the list. I wanted to scream, but a twelve-year-old boy is supposed to be very cool about such matters.

The final cut was coming up in a few days, so I was extremely nervous, wondering if I would be on the fifteen-man roster. During all this, I managed to maintain a decent grade point average, but I don't know how. My whole life was centered around getting on this basketball team. Finally, the list came out, and Coach posted the fifteen members of the seventh-grade basketball team on the field house door. Once again, I went through the same anxieties I had for the first cut. I started reading the names from the top, and once again, I felt my heart sink with each name, and there it was. I made the team!

I was so happy I could hardly contain my emotions. This made me feel like a big shot on campus. I had taken a blood test about a week before the team was announced, and I wasn't too concerned about the results. There was no such thing as home monitoring of blood sugar in those days, at least, not to my knowledge. I took a blood test about once every couple of months. I assumed all the bad news from this disease was out, and I wouldn't have to worry about anything else. When the results came back, my doctor wasn't satisfied, so he asked me to quit the basketball team.

After all my hard work, this was such devastating news. There I was in the same circumstance I was in during football season. I started to ask God why he was doing this to me. Because it was clear he was punishing me.

My seventh-grade year continued without much fanfare. I was still very disappointed that I couldn't play basketball that year. I knew track season was coming up, but I really wasn't that enthused about track. I did get some encouraging news from my doctor. Apparently, my blood sugar was at a level where he would allow me to be a part of the track team.

My brother Cedric had taught me at an early age how to run hurdles, so that's where I concentrated my efforts in track and field. I was never the fastest hurdler at my school, but I did have the best form, and I looked really good while running the hurdles. I did manage to place and score points in many of the track meets in which we competed. Being a part of the track team was a rewarding experience. In fact, it was the only sport I was consistently a part of throughout junior high and high school, every single year after that. It never seemed to fill the void of not being a part of the football or basketball teams that year.

HOMECOMING

When my eighth-grade year began, there was lots of excitement for me since my doctor had cleared me to play football. The prior year, I didn't feel as if I mattered much at my school because I didn't play football, but now that I was on the team, it gave me a sense of importance among my peers. I picked up where I left off in seventh grade before I quit the team. I was on the first team as a split end, and I was the second team quarterback.

In my opinion, I was a good split end, but our offensive scheme didn't allow the split end to get the ball very much. We had big running backs and a big quarterback, so our offensive philosophy was to run the ball every play. The coaches called it "three yards and a cloud of dust." We would seldom even practice a pass play in which I would get the ball as a receiver. Although this was the case, I persevered, thinking, at some point, I would get an opportunity to show my talents as a receiver.

As the second team quarterback, I had plenty of opportunity to control the ball. Unfortunately, I had to practice against the first team defense. We were basically glorified tackling dummies for the first team defense. It seemed as if every time I took a snap as the second team quarterback, I got buried in the dirt. For some reason, I didn't mind the torture because it gave me a since of bravado, and it garnered a great deal of respect among my teammates and the coaches.

As a receiver in our offensive philosophy of run the ball at all times, my main job on every play was to go down field and block. I made it my mission to be the best down field blocker I could be. In our first game that year, we played Mount Pleasant, which was the same team that beat us in the district championship the year before.

They beat us 36 to 8 in this game. The loss was quite embarrassing to say the least. A few days after the loss, a group of us, along with our coach, were discussing what happened in the game, and I mentioned out of everything that happened, I did my job of going downfield to block. Later on, we had a meeting with the whole team, and my coach called me out for saying I did my job. He didn't call my name, but we both knew who he was talking about. My coach made it very clear to me that my attitude was quite selfish after such a demeaning loss. I learned a great lesson in humility in that sequence of events.

I felt as if I had lost much of the respect I had gained from that coach with the statement "I did my job," and I would spend the rest of my junior high and high school years trying to regain his respect.

Eight grade went along with no major events. We went through the daily grind of practice. Every once in a while, they would throw me a pass in practice, and this would keep my hopes up for possible game time receptions, but it never came to fruition. One week in practice, the second team offense had to run the opposing team's offense. The opposing team was running the option. No one on our team was familiar with this concept, except me. My brother Cedric had taught me well on running the option. As the second team quarterback, I ran it almost to perfection, and the first team defense didn't have a clue of how to stop it. This didn't make me a starting quarterback, but I think it did solidify my position as a back-up quarterback for the rest of my years in junior high and high school.

I finally graduated from junior high school with no great accolades, but I was happy to be moving on to high school. Most people, when making the transition from junior high to high school, it can be a bit overwhelming. For our freshman class, it was an easy transition, mostly because of our success athletically in junior high. Many of the upper classmen showed great respect for our accomplishments.

The difference between junior high and high school was in junior high, we were told what courses we would take. But in high school, we had some input in the courses we would take. There were many courses we were required to take, but we had options when choosing electives. Many of the boys in my school would take agricultural courses, while many of the girls would take homemaking courses. Many boys would take homemaking courses just to meet and build relationships with the girls. While I admit, I did take one homemaking course during my high school career, but most of my electives consisted of courses like speech, business, Spanish, and health occupations. When I would reveal the courses I was taking to my classmates, they would look at me sideways because my choices were so nonconventional.

Football was different in high school because we started practice two weeks before the school year, and it was extremely hot. Another difference was two-a-day practice during the first two weeks. For those of you who are not familiar with this term, it's when you practice once in the morning and once in the afternoon. Everyone had an opportunity to play football in our class, but two-a-day practice would discourage many from ever putting on pads again. It was difficult, but for me, I never felt as if I had a choice. No amount of pain or suffering would dissuade me from my destination of becoming a great football player.

There were many things to hate about two-a-day practice, but the thing I dreaded the most was the rope maze. This thing stood about ten inches off the ground and was constructed of a one-inch-diameter pipe frame. The frame was about ten yards long, and at every yard along the width of the frame was a rope crossing the frame with one rope running lengthwise, along the center of the frame. We did several drills with the rope maze, but what I hated was when we had to sprint through the maze. The first time I did it, I tripped over a rope. Every subsequent time I did it, I would trip. I would have all kinds of cuts and bruises from the falls. Every time I ran through, I would trip and fall, aggravating the same cuts and bruises. Eventually, I would learn how to run through the maze without tripping, but it was very frustrating in the beginning.

My freshman year was about the same as junior high in football. I was the first team split end and the second team quarterback on the freshman team. We ran the ball all the time, so there weren't many passes coming my way in games. I do think I regained some respect from my coach, who, despite my medical condition, saw a never-give-up attitude in the way I hustled in practice. My never quit attitude continued through all sports, and I developed a bit of a reputation as a leader among my teammates in all sports.

Sophomore year started as usual with two-a-day practice. All the freshman from the previous year moved up to the junior varsity team. I was still the first team split end and the second team quarterback, but coaches were encouraging me to concentrate most of my efforts in becoming a better quarterback. I didn't understand why I was receiving this encouragement until about four games into the season, when our first team quarterback was moved up to the varsity team, and I replaced him as the first team quarterback on the junior varsity team. It was a huge surprise to me, but I gladly accepted the challenge. It was an opportunity to become the football star that had seemed to be eluding me in previous years.

I had been the second team quarterback for several years, so the playbook was not an issue. But execution with the first team was where I needed work. I had one week of practice to get all the timing down with the first team. By the time of the next game, I felt very comfortable in my ability to run the offense as the starting quarterback.

As game day came, I was extremely excited for this new opportunity. I got some great news the morning of the game. My oldest brother, Joc, was going to be in town, and he would be attending the game. Joc had never seen me play, so it was a wonderful surprise. I would remember the excitement of going to his games, but I didn't remember actually seeing him play. Knowing he would be there just gave me added confidence.

The game was against Paul Pewitt High School. It started as our games usually do. We ran the ball virtually every play. Our first drive was going quite well. We were moving the ball, and Paul Pewitt's defense couldn't stop our offense. We were moving down the field, until coach called a quarterback sneak. I was so excited about my first rush coming up. When the ball was snapped, I immediately leaned into the center and pushed forward. I felt hands tugging on me trying to pull me to the ground, but they didn't have much success. I was slowly gaining yardage as I moved through the scrum of defenders. Little did I realize one of the defenders was pulling the ball out of my hands while I was moving forward. So the drive stalled after I recorded my first fumble. It was quite embarrassing, and it was the last time in the game in which coach allowed me to run the football.

Fortunately, Paul Pewitt's offense was not very effective against our defense, so they weren't able to capitalize on my mistake. We got the ball back, and after a long drive, we scored a touchdown to go ahead six to zero. On the extra point, I was surprised when my coach called a pass play, especially after I fumbled the ball on the earlier drive. The play was called eighteen bootleg pass. I had to roll out to the right and pass to the tight end as he runs a quick five and out. The play was a success, and it was my first and only completion of the game. I completed 100 percent of my passes that night. A perfect completion rate! This made the score 8 to 0.

The rest of the game was a back and forth defensive struggle. I ended up running the ball three more times for twenty-eight yards in the last series to run out the clock. All three rushes were busted plays, and I really wasn't supposed to have the ball, but it worked out. The final score was 8 to 0. I had won my first game as the starting quarterback, and the team was very proud of what we were able to accomplish.

I was eager to spend the rest of the season as the starting quarterback, but then, diabetes would rear its ugly head again. My doctor informed me I would have to quit playing football once again. It was devastating to know that for a second time in my life, I would have to quit playing football because of diabetes. I was hoping as I became more familiar with the disease I would be better prepared to deal with the disease.

The football season ended with no significant consequences. I watched the final two games from the bench as my teammates moved on without me. Such an incredible opportunity ends in disappointment, and there was nothing I could do about it. My only hope for the rest of my sophomore year was basketball and track. I continued to make every effort within my power to get ready for the upcoming basketball season.

The news from my doctor was very positive, so he allowed me to play basketball and run track for the rest of the year. Although I didn't get to complete the football season, it was some consolation to compete in the other sports for the remainder of the school year.

As my junior year was quickly approaching, I spent the summer working out as best I knew how. I went running on the blacktop road near my house every day. I probably weighed in at 140 pounds as a junior and stood about five feet, nine inches tall. I didn't really stand out in the size department. This was the first year I would have to compete with upper classmen for playing time. Once the football season started with two-a-day practices, it seemed the coaches wanted me to play quarterback exclusively. In my mind, I didn't think I could ever see playing time as quarterback, but I felt I could compete with the upper classmen at split end. The coaches didn't allow me to play split end, so I went along with the program and concentrated on the second team quarterback position.

Most people would consider the second team quarterback as a glorified hitting dummy because he is up against the first team defense. The second team lineman had good intentions but could never contain the first team defense. Practice became a daily ritual of my body getting pounded into the ground. It had become such a routine that I had forgotten my dreams of becoming a star. My focus was to survive each day of practice.

The first scrimmage game came with much anticipation as most of us juniors on the team were new to varsity football. We went to Carthage, Texas, for that game. The first team ran through their series of plays without much success, but when the second team took the field, we moved the ball with great consistency. We even managed to score a touchdown. The first scrimmage was a triumph for the second team, and I felt good about our contribution to the team.

The second scrimmage was equally exciting since it was against one of our staunch rivals, the Atlanta Rabbits. Practice during that week was about the same as usual, except I was optimistic because of our success in the last game. Once the game started, our first team was still not very successful in their series of downs, but when the second team took the field, we picked up where we left off in the last game. We moved the ball very well, and I threw a touchdown pass to end the last drive. My position as the second team quarterback seemed to be promising as the season began.

We were about to go into our first regular season game in Idabel, Oklahoma. As the second team quarterback, I wasn't expected to get in the game, but I was ready if needed. It was a tough defensive battle, and we were down 12 to 8 in the fourth quarter when our starting quarterback went down with an injury. I thought to myself, this will be my opportunity to become the star. I began to warm up on the sideline because I thought I would be going into the game, but the coaches had a different plan. They decided to allow a much bigger and stronger player to go in as quarterback. This player had mainly played running back and linebacker on defense in practice, but he never played quarterback in practice. He was a senior and an outstanding athlete who was destined to go on to bigger and better things in football. I was crushed that the coaches didn't think enough of my ability to allow me to go into the game when our starting quarterback went down. We lost the game, and I didn't know what my future was.

To this point in my life, I had devoted everything to football. My understanding was the second team quarterback would play when the starting quarterback went down. The whole weekend I had to question my entire existence. The week earlier, the junior varsity quarterback had suffered a broken arm, so the following Monday, the coaches informed me I would be moving down to junior varsity to play quarterback. They felt this would give me some game experience that would help me for the following year. The junior varsity played on Thursdays, so the coaches would allow me to play on Thursdays and dress on Fridays with the varsity.

This wasn't the best situation for my football career, but I was having fun getting to play and having great success in the process. During this time, I was very much an all-American teenage boy, and girls were becoming a major priority, and football was taking a back seat. But I always felt it was a means to impress the girls. There was one girl in particular that I admired from afar since middle school. In my naive backwoods mentality, I considered her the most beautiful girl who ever existed. In those days, all I had to offer was reasonably good looks and my status as an athlete. She really didn't stand out other than being a natural beauty in our town. These superficial attributes seemed to bring the two of us together.

By this time, I had my driver's license, but my sister, Carlotta who was a senior, didn't have a driver's license. This scenario made things quite awkward because I wanted to use my mother's car to go see my girlfriend, but I was the designated chauffeur for Carlotta and my cousins who lived down the road from us. I never considered how selfish I was thinking that life was so unfair when I had to drive my sister and cousins around instead of spending time with my girlfriend. My sister and cousins were very attractive girls, so guys would flock to the car when we were together. And I'm sure the girls enjoyed this attention, but I was miserable.

On some occasion, I would have the opportunity to go and spend time with my girlfriend, but it was never enough. When we did spend time together, it was extremely awkward. I'm not sure how she felt, but my heart raced at a mile a minute when we were together. My palms were sweaty, and I had no idea what to say to her. At school, we would walk up and down the hallways together and probably wouldn't say five words to each other. We had very little in common. We barely spoke, and we hardly ever looked at each other. But I thought I was in heaven.

Finally, we made it to homecoming, and I had a date who everyone at school considered my girlfriend. I bought her a corsage, and she was devastatingly beautiful that night. I played with the junior varsity football team that Thursday, so I had the option to dress with the varsity for the homecoming game. Instead of dressing with the varsity team, I chose to spend that evening with my girlfriend. My mother had planned for my sister and cousins to have rides for the evening, so I could spend most of my time with my girl. The only problem was after the game, she and I would have to give my mother a ride home. Everything was fine that evening, except on the way, taking my mother home, we had a flat tire. I had no idea how to change a tire at the time, but two of my cousins saw us on the side of the road and stopped to help. I probably didn't impress my girlfriend with my lack of mechanical skills, but we did get the flat changed and got back on the road.

We dropped my mother off at home, and I drove my date home. We said goodnight to each other without so much as a handshake. I was too afraid to attempt to kiss her goodnight. Our relationship would fizzle out a couple of weeks after homecoming. I think I put her on a pedestal and worshipped her rather than treated her as a fellow human. I was really hurt after the break up, but I always had football.

The season went on like clockwork. I continued to play with the junior varsity on Thursdays and dress with the varsity on Friday. Around the middle of the season, the starting junior varsity quarterback's broken arm healed, so I was allowed to play split end on the junior varsity. This was a major turning point in my football career. The coaches were taking notice of my qualities as a receiver as I had become a serious deep threat scoring touchdowns in each of the last three games. My work at the end of the season on the junior varsity as a split end had solidified my position as the starting varsity split end for the next year. It seemed as though my dreams of becoming a football star were back on track once again.

NOT COOL

High school is an awkward period for most teenagers, and for me, there was no exception. Looking back, you might say I was admired by most in my peer group. I worked at Marion County Hospital as an orderly on the weekends. I was on the student council. I was a decent student, although I didn't put much effort into school and study. I was an officer in the Fellowship of Christian Athletes, and I played multiple sports. Even with all these accolades, I was still a goofy, insecure teenager. I would question if I was big enough, or tall enough, or smart enough, or good-looking enough among other things.

When football season ended during my junior year in high school, I had to make a decision on, if I was going to play basketball or use that winter to get ready for track. A friend of mine, who was one of the best hurdlers in the nation at the, time decided not to play basketball, so I decided to follow him and not play basketball. My training methods probably weren't as good as they could've been, but I did what I knew to do, and that was run. All my free time was spent running at the track or running on the road.

Although I didn't play basketball for the team, I somehow managed to play in pickup games around town at every opportunity. In retrospect, I think I should've played basketball on the team my junior year. Every morning during my junior year, when I got to school, guys would meet in the gym to play basketball, and I was in the center of it all. One day during the Christmas break, I was at the gym playing basketball while the basketball team was getting ready to go play a game on the road. I guess, due to the holidays, they were missing a few players, so the coach at the time asked me if I would go with them and play that night. Had I chosen to play that night,

I think I would've been a part of the team for the rest of the season. I chose not to play, and the decision somewhat solidified my high school basketball career, or lack thereof.

I continued to work out to get ready for track, while playing basketball and dreaming of football stardom. It was an excruciating offseason with no events to compete at and no crowds cheering. It was just work, and I really didn't care for the work, but I managed to struggle through till the beginning of track season.

The season started like any other season with the Wiley College Relays. I think, every year through junior high and high school, we started track season at the Wiley College Relays, and every year, it was always cold and rainy. This year, the temperature was about thirty degrees, and on and off sleet. The weather was so bad we were the only high school to show up along with a few individuals from the Wiley Colleges track team. We ended up competing in a few events, until they finally canceled the rest of the meet. I can definitely say it wasn't a very successful start to the track season.

The next few weeks were spent competing against much larger schools, where we were basically outmatched in every event. Fortunately, it would prepare us to compete with schools of comparable size and the schools within our district. By the time we started to compete in our district, we were winning the meets or finishing second.

The turning point in the season was a weekend where we had a meet on Friday in Jacksonville, Texas, and Saturday in Linden-Kildare, Texas. When we got to Jacksonville on Friday, I knew it was going to be another typical meet, where we were out matched by the bigger schools, but everyone was there, competing as best we could. After a rough day of not much success, we had a long travel night back home to Jefferson, and the thought of having to get up to do it again the next morning at Linden-Kildare was exhausting to think about.

The next morning, I was drained as well as my teammates, both physically and mentally, but we gathered up enough strength to make it back to school and get on the bus to make the trip. At this meet, we were one of the favorites to win because all the schools competing were about our size or smaller. It was a beautiful early spring day, where the sun was shining and not a cloud in the sky. When we got there our 4×100-meter relay team began to warm up. This particular day, I ran the third leg of the relay. We won our heat and had the second fastest time in the preliminaries, which got us a very good lane for the finals that afternoon.

My next event was the 110-meter hurdles. There was no way I could ever win this event, but I had the opportunity to score in the top six or get a medal in the top three. I was in the second of three preliminary heats of the race. I watched the first heat in great anticipation for my chance to run.

When I got in the starting blocks for my heat, I was very nervous as usual, but I gathered enough composure to settle down and run the race. When the starter shot the gun, I was off with the crowd and probably ahead of the crowd. Over the first few hurdles, I was running well, and I had a slight lead over everyone in the race. At about the eighth hurdle, the most embarrassing thing you could ever imagine happened to me. I lost complete control of my bowel muscles and defecated all over myself. I finished the race and won the heat. My time was good enough to get me into the finals, but that wasn't my concern at the time. You talk about a nightmare for an insecure teenager. I had excrement all over myself. The only thing I was wearing was a jock strap and my uniform shorts, and both were an utter mess.

After the race, I rushed to the closest restroom to try and clean up a bit, but supplies for that sort thing were limited. And I didn't have a change of clothes, so I walked around the rest of the day, smelling like a pig in a pigsty. I couldn't clean up much, and I still had another preliminary event to run in before the morning was over. I competed in the 200-meter dash and made it to the finals in that event also. Early in the day, I could barely smell the stench secreting from my body, but as the day went on, the aroma got stronger to me. I can only imagine what others were thinking when they came within a few feet of me. I even tried to put my warmup on over my uniform to hide the smell from others, but I don't think I was fooling anyone.

For the rest of the day, I walked around with my head down, and I continued to compete as best I could under the circumstances. No one said anything to me about the situation I found myself in, neither did anyone make fun of me, which high school kids would tend to do. But I could imagine people were talking. I did well in my estimation in all my events that afternoon. We got second place in the 4×100-meter relay. I got third place in the 110-meter hurdles, and I got fourth place in the 200-meter dash, although many people felt I got third place in that event. It was the most successful day I had ever had in track, but it was also probably the most embarrassing day of my life.

On the ride back to Jefferson on the bus, I had two awards in my hand, but I really couldn't celebrate with my teammates because of the stench that was resonating from my body. I tried to get myself as far away from others on the bus as I could to no avail. The scent was so strong I could hardly stand myself. No one ever spoke to me about what happened that day, but I wonder if anyone, my teammates or anyone I competed against, ever discussed or made fun of me about that day.

Despite the horrendous incident at the track meet, I was very optimistic about my future in track after my success that day. I heard from many people at school talking about how well I did, and I was a bit full of myself. There were only a few weeks left in the track season, so I continued training everyday as usual and looked forward to the district track meet.

I thought my diabetes was well under control during track season, but one day, I had a major insulin reaction. It wasn't very common for me, but my prior experiences suggested I would recover soon after. Unfortunately, things didn't turn out so well. After the reaction, I was able to function normally at school, but at track practice, I was extremely lifeless and lethargic. This was evident in my lack of ability to train, and in the times I was recording in my events. They were much slower than normal. At this point in the season, when you should see significant improvement, I was declining exponentially.

As the season progressed, I never got back to the level I achieved at the Linden-Kildare track meet. I never consulted my physician about the situation thinking I would be able to lift myself out of the physical cellar I found myself in. When I think of this episode in my life, I often wonder if the loose bowl incident had something to do with my subsequent insulin reaction, and the ultimate decline of my ability that so abruptly took over my life at the time.

The season went on, and I tried to compete, but I never got through the lifeless lethargic feeling I had after the insulin reaction. The district track meet came, and I was basically a nonfactor, not even making it to the finals in any of my events. It was a very disappointing time, but my level of optimism was never swayed as I looked forward to the future.

As my junior year of high school was winding down, I reflected on the triumphs and disappointments of the year and some of the decisions made. Disappointed that I was relegated back to the junior varsity football team, but pleased with my performance. I was very pleased with what I accomplished at the Linden-Kildare track meet, but the rest of the track season was a letdown. During the awards ceremony, at the end of the year, I received two awards—one for football and one for track. In retrospect, I think I would've played basketball my junior year because, now, I look back on that time with some regret for not achieving my full potential that year.

As the summer of 1980 rolled around, I had to start thinking about my future and what I would do after high school. The reality was sinking in that I may not be the football star I wanted to be, although I hadn't totally given up on the dream completely. I knew of Kilgore College, near Jefferson, so I started thinking if I can't get a scholarship to play football, I would go there. My sister, Carlotta, who graduated from high school in 1980 decided to go to Kilgore College to study photography. I think she decided to go there, based on some of the discussions I was having with our mother about the school. I don't think she was ever really committed to the idea of going to Kilgore.

During the summer, I continued to work part-time at Marion County Hospital as an orderly. I got the job through the health occupations class I was taking at school. I never really aspired to do anything in the healthcare field, but had I had a more big-picture mentality, who knows. I probably could be a physician right now. I didn't have many big-picture ideas in those days other than becoming a famous football player. It seemed almost like each day was a million years, and I would always be in that little town of Jefferson, Texas. The future was so far away I didn't have to concern myself with it for a long time to come.

I was working out on occasion during the summer, getting ready for my upcoming senior year of football. I was also receiving some correspondence from the Texas Rehabilitation Commission about them, helping me with tuition and books after high school based on my diabetes, which they considered a disability. I wasn't too familiar with the financial aspects of going to college. All I knew was that all my brothers and sisters went to college after high school, so I just assumed that's what you were supposed to do. Never really considering any strain it would put on my parents financially.

Two of my brothers, Joc and Cedric, worked as draftsman, and I had shown great ability to draw freehand while growing up, so I decided to study drafting and design technology when I would go to college. It seemed like a logical choice, and it was something I enjoyed doing. I was feeling pretty good about some of my future plans and what the future would hold for me.

SUPERSTAR

The summer was coming to an end and two-a-day practice was about to start for my senior year of football. I was extremely excited about this season because of the success I had achieved the previous year as a wide receiver on the junior varsity team. It was apparent the coaches were going to use me and another one of my teammates to shuttle in plays, so I would be splitting time with him at wide receiver. Even though we were splitting time, it was established early that I would be the main focus at wide receiver. Despite my getting more attention from the coaches at receiver, it was evident our offensive philosophy wasn't changing. It was always run the ball at all cost. Every so often, they would through me a pass in practice, and it was just enough to get my hopes up.

Typically, you want to stand by the adage that practice makes perfect, so I would think a team would practice a play they felt confident in almost at nauseam, until they perfected it. This is what we did for most of our running plays but passing plays that involved me were ran sparingly. I probably didn't possess the diva mentality, most professional wide receivers have, or I would've spoke up to coaches and said "Give me the ball." Instead, I lurked in the background and hoped for things to change.

We started the season with two scrimmage games at the end of the summer. Both of those games resulted in not a single pass being thrown in my direction. My frustration was building, but I've always been one to persevere through difficult times. The first real game of the season was against Daingerfield, and we had to prepare for them. We also had to choose jersey numbers before the game. In previous years, I always wore jersey numbers in the tens because of my time at quarterback. If I was playing wide receiver, it didn't make much difference if I had a number in the tens.

Because of my success the previous year, I had adopted the nick-name Sean Swann from some of my teammates. This year, I decided to wear the number 88 to emulate the famous Pittsburg Steeler wide receiver, Lynn Swann. Fridays, at school, we were allowed to wear our jerseys to help build school moral during the day of the game. I've always been very particular about uniforms and how they look. Our team wore the same uniforms as the year before, but among all the high schools I had seen, I felt we had the sharpest uniforms. And I thought I looked very good in number 88.

Daingerfield was a home game for us, and they were somewhat of a rival. And everybody in Jefferson was at the game. There was an excitement throughout the stadium that night. The first half was spent trading scores. Daingerfield scored two touchdowns, and we scored two touchdowns. The score was 14 to 14. Our two scores were made by one of my teammates, our tight end, who scored on two long passes. While I was happy that we were competing, but I was a bit jealous of my teammate because he was getting all these passes. And the coaches didn't bother to throw the ball in my direction.

The second half was a defensive battle, where neither team scored until Daingerfield kicked a field goal to score with a minute and thirty seconds left in the game to take the lead at 17 to 14. When we got the ball back, time was running out for us. As I stood next to my coaches, waiting for the next play to take in, they were discussing what we should do when one coach suggested we should run a split end screen where I would catch the ball and throw it down field to our tight end. Immediately, my heart started to race. This is a play we had never ran in practice. Also, I hadn't caught a pass in a game set-ting since the prior year, and with the game on the line, they wanted to put the game in my hands.

After the discussion, the coaches had agreed to run the play. Being the hero in the clutch moment of a big game was always my desire, but I was still in disbelief the coaches would trust me in this situation. I ran to the huddle and told our quarterback, the play. He then relayed the play to everyone else in the huddle. We broke the huddle, and everyone ran to their position. The quarterback sounded out the cadences before the snap of the ball, and I was so anxious knowing the ball was coming to me. When the ball snapped, I took a step forward to force the defensive back, covering me to take a step back. Then I took two steps behind the line of scrimmage, and the ball was already on its way to me. My thought was *I have to catch this ball.* I caught the ball, and my next step was to position my body to throw the ball down field.

As I repositioned my body to throw the ball, I could feel the defense bearing down on me, so I had to get rid of it as quickly as possible. I saw the tight end running down field, and I threw the ball as far as I could. When I let go of the ball, someone on the defense hit me, and I went to the ground. While on the ground, all I could see were the home bleachers. I didn't see the tight end catch the ball, but I did see the crowd in the bleachers erupt with jubilation. He did catch the ball and ultimately scored a touchdown on the play. Here I am, a senior in high school, and my childhood dream has finally come to fruition. I am a hero! People talked about that play for days on end. Slowly, the feeling of euphoria faded away in our community, but the feeling is always present in my heart and mind, as if it happened yesterday.

We ran that play maybe three more times during the season, never running it in practice, but without the same success. Our season continued without much fanfare. Each week came and went to a point, where they all ran together. Sometimes, I would get a pass thrown to me, but not enough to get any college scouts interested. I wasn't considered a threat at all to opposing teams.

Overall, our team was reasonably successful that year. We were seven and two going into the last game. It was about time for me to face the fact I wasn't going to go on and play football in college, but my never-give-up attitude wouldn't allow me to set the dream aside. It was evident when the next fall semester would come around, I would be studying drafting, so I started to prepare for another career.

At our last football game of the season, our team had an opportunity. If we won, we would be eligible for the state playoffs. If we lost our season, my high school football career would be over. It was a cold and misty night in New Boston, Texas, and we were playing the New Boston Lions. On paper, it seemed to be a winnable game, but we would have to play well. Nothing for our team went right that night, and it was an extremely lackluster performance for us. I had one opportunity to catch a pass that night on a slant across the middle. The pass was high, but I should've caught it. Instead, the ball bounced off my hands, and it was intercepted. That was the last time I touched the football in my high school football career. We lost the game by the score of 20 to 7, and that was it for me and football.

It was a long ride home, but I was already looking forward to playing basketball to occupy my time. Our basketball team wasn't projected to be one of the better teams in our district, but I thought I would be an integral part of whatever the team might be. I ended up spending most of my time on the bench. Like most competitive people, I thought I should have gotten more playing time, instead I was sort of a malcontent and a subtle disruption to anything my coach was trying to accomplish. Basketball started and ended, and before I realized it, I was over halfway through my senior year.

Track season was quickly approaching, and I was excited about what I might be able to accomplish this year. I was always a hurdler, but I felt I could compete in many of the sprints such as the 200 meters and the 400 meters. The previous year, I had a brief period of success, so I thought it would carry over to this year. I would score points in my individual events, but I never stood out as one of the true stars on our team. Regardless of the choices I made—whether to be a full-time quarterback or to play wide receiver, whether to play basketball, or the events I chose to compete in track—I had to face the fact I was a very average athlete. It's nothing wrong with being an average athlete and loving to play lots of sports or watching sports on television. A guy I use to play basketball with at a community center called himself a "weekend warrior," and I adopted that name for myself.

The track season came to an end, and I was looking at graduation. It was time for a new chapter in my life.

That summer after graduation, my friend and I decided to go to Kilgore to look for housing since we both were going to school there.

The dorms were filled, so we had to find housing elsewhere. We eventually found a place known in Kilgore called the Rock House. It was owned by the pastor of a church right next door to the house. It had the name Rock House because of the rock facade around the building, which matched the church. My friend got a room by himself, and I got a roommate.

When the semester was about to start, I was packing and getting ready to move to Kilgore. I always looked to my mother and father for whatever I needed, but my mother told me if I ever found myself in need of anything, I should go to God. When she said this, it made me realize I won't be able to depend on her forever, but I can always reach out to my God for wisdom and guidance. This made a profound impact on my life, and it gave me a new perspective on life from the one I had growing up. I knew of a Heavenly Father, but I didn't have a real relationship with him.

DREAMS DIFFERED

There were an assortment of characters living in the Rock House with me. Everyone living there was a student at Kilgore College, except for a guy who we called Notto. Notto was from Cuba and spoke very little English. He was sort of the overseer of the house, although we didn't answer to him at all. There was my roommate, Karl, who was from a small town near Jefferson. I would describe Karl as extremely quick-witted. There was Greg and his cousin, Shank. These guys were the best dressed and coolest of the group. There was Terry, who was the typical hardworking student. All Terry ever did was work, go to class, and take an occasional nap. Then there was Jesse, another small-town boy, whom you would swear he fell off a turnip truck he was so country.

My first semester at Kilgore was just getting a feel for the college routine and all that entailed. This consisted of making sure I knew where classes were, learning all the shortcuts around campus, and identifying all the women on campus. I settled in fairly easily, and before long, it felt like I was at home. The only thing missing was sports the way I knew it in junior high and high school. Fortunately, we had intramural sports, and I became very involved.

During the fall, we played flag football. It wasn't quite what I was used to, but I loved the game. There were no crowds where people were cheering, but it did provide a means to play. I'm sure I took it more seriously than most who played, but I still felt I was destined for the NFL. Most of the guys from the Rock House played on a team together, and we were pretty good. But we could've been better if we didn't have all the egos to deal with. Mine was probably one of the bigger egos, although I wasn't one to express it. I mostly played quarterback, but occasionally, I would play receiver. We didn't win any championships, but everyone thought we were the team to beat.

All the guys who lived in the Rock House did everything together. On Thursday nights and Saturday nights, we would go to all the clubs in the nearby towns. I think people saw us as a group when we went places together. You can say we were all each other's wing man.

Within our Rock House group, we had several subgroups. My subgroup consisted of myself and my roommate Karl. Sometimes, my friend from Jefferson was a part of our subgroup, but it was mostly Karl and me. I had a car when I first started at Kilgore, but one day, while I was driving to a flag football game, the car caught on fire. I was reduced to a bunch of walking around campus at this point, but Karl had a car. In fact, Karl introduced me to driving a standard shift vehicle.

There was something about Karl that girls liked, so this afforded me opportunities I didn't normally have with the opposite sex. I had to be on my toes with Karl because of his quick wit. He was always trying to find situations to embarrass you. There was one time when he and I went out with these three very attractive girls. Of course, I was very attracted to one of these girls. While we were out, a guy asked our group, "Which one isn't with you?"

Karl quickly pointed to me and said, "This one."

It was funny to everyone in our vicinity, and I was completely embarrassed. I wasn't Karl's only target for embarrassment, for he shared it equally around the Rock House, so I didn't take it too personally.

The first semester at Kilgore was quite an experience for me. In my sheltered upbringing, I had never partied or dated or hung out with the guys as much as I did that first semester. Through all that, I felt the need to constantly read the Bible. For some reason, I felt the importance of the Bible, even though I didn't quite understand what I was reading. I would revert back to the conversation I had with my mom when she told me to seek God when I find myself in need.

As the semester was closing, I had pretty well established myself as a student, but I still had other dreams not yet fulfilled. I was going back to my high school to speak with my coaches about film they could send to the coaches at Kilgore, so they could possibly take a look at my ability as a football player. Nothing ever came of that, but I continued to be hopeful. The next semester was slowly approaching, and there was an opening in the dorms. Karl had decided to join the navy during the next semester, so I knew he wouldn't be my roommate anymore. But my friend from Jefferson decided to take the dorm opening with me.

The second semester was somewhat routine, except for this girl I met. Her name was Janet Sweet, and her name described her beauty. She was slightly overweight, but somehow, she carried it quite well. And she had eyes that were extremely hypnotizing. Something told me she was out of my league, but I constantly felt her eyes piercing my soul. And I knew she was interested in me. Immediately, after we started to date, my status around campus began to rise. The guys wanted to be in my position, and the girls wanted to be with me.

Being a hopeless romantic, one of my goals in life was to meet a beautiful girl, fall in love, and live happily ever after. I thought Janet had fulfilled my dreams, and all was well. Janet was very opportunistic, and she had a bit of a wild side. I was considered one of the good guys, but I was so mesmerized by her I began to adapt to some of her influences. It was clear that Janet's way of life was too fast for my "country boy" taste, but I was so beguiled that I was willing to hang on at all cost.

We continued to date through the semester, and our relationship lasted through the summer. During the summer, my mom allowed me to drive her car one weekend to Palestine, where Janet lived and spend the weekend with her and her family. There was nothing special about the weekend, but for me, it was life-changing at the time. I thought it solidified our relationship for the future. Janet gave me a framed 8"×10" photo of herself that I considered quite provocative. In the photo, she was lying down, and she had on a maroon jumpsuit with cowboy boots and a cowboy hat. I looked forward to telling everyone back home the girl in the picture was my girlfriend. I spent the rest of the summer dreaming of mine and Janet's life together.

When the next semester started, I was ready to be in a relationship with Janet, but when we got back to school, she was very distant. Finally, she told me she wasn't comfortable in the relationship, and we should, maybe, take a break. She asked me to give back to her the picture she had given me. I gave the picture back, trying to give the impression that I really didn't care about what we had. Deep inside, I was devastated. My heart was broken once again, and my world had come to an end. I had learned later that Janet was dating a guy on the Kilgore basketball team. We would see each other on campus, and we would speak as if we shared nothing. It was all I could do to keep from falling at her feet when I saw her and begging her to take me back.

I felt like I was giving the impression that I was so over my relationship with Janet. One day, she and I talked, and she told me that I had reverted back to the shell (I never knew people thought I was in a shell) I was in before we started dating. All the time I thought my facade gave the impression I was doing OK, but Janet could see my hurt. And I wonder if everyone else could see it. Eventually, there were other girls at Kilgore that I dated, but I would've dropped them all to be with Janet. In retrospect, I suppose I was fortunate she broke up with me because she was changing me, and not for the better.

Life went on at Kilgore College, and between trying to hook up with different girls and going to class every day, nothing could separate me from my athletic pursuits. I organized a very successful intramural flag football team that I thought could win the championship, until I allowed all the guys from the Rock House to become a part of my team with their inflated egos. The season ended in pure disaster, all because I didn't stick to my convictions of staying with the team I had originally put together. Not winning a championship didn't mean that much to me. Being able to compete was thrilling enough. For me, it was always about participating rather than winning. This was probably to my detriment as an athlete. The killer instinct was never part of my personality.

I also managed to put an intramural basketball team together that was very competitive. We weren't expected to win a championship with that team, but other teams were aware of how good we were. They didn't take us lightly when they played us. We won more games than we lost, and the games we lost were barnburners. Once again, the wins and losses didn't matter as much to me as the opportunity to play the game.

After all the intramural sports were over, there wasn't much left for organized competition. My friends and I would play pickup basketball every chance we got, or just through the football around the yard. I even played a lot of tennis during my time at Kilgore, even though I wasn't the best tennis player. I had a group of friends who I use to wake early in the mornings to go run, and they were very resentful of my persistence in waking them for our two-mile runs. I would find something to do athletically wherever I was. I think my diabetes always gave a drive to compete with people who didn't have a problem like that, just to prove I could compete regardless of my disability.

As the second semester of that year was coming to a close, most of the students who started at Kilgore College with me in the fall of 1981 were contemplating graduation. The reality of this milestone didn't escape my thought process either. I did have a plan of what I was going to do after high school, but my plan after Kilgore was quite vague. Most of all, I wanted to get a job within my field of study, but drafting jobs weren't exactly falling off trees. My other option was to just find a job. Eventually, we made it to graduation, and many people were on pins and needles because no one knew their final grades, and there was a rumor going around when they passed out degrees at graduation. The degrees were placed in a beautifully bound leather book. If you didn't pass, it would be a blank piece of paper in your book, and if you did pass, your degree would be placed in the book. Fortunately, my degree was inside my book, and I completed my course of study at the end of two years at Kilgore College.

I was quite diligent in my quest to find employment after graduation, but it was a slow process. I tried to find drafting jobs, but it didn't seem like anything was available. I finally found a job at a restaurant called Bonanza in Marshall, Texas. I had never worked in a restaurant in my life, but they were willing to give me an opportunity. After I got hired, my sister Carlotta applied for a job at Bonanza, and she was hired there also. We worked together for a couple of months. I eventually got a job at K-Bobs restaurant in Marshall, Texas. They gave me a slight raise and a bit more responsibility.

My father helped me get a car, so I was able to get around on my own. Life had become routine. I went to work, and I went home. I did manage to get involved with a city league basketball team, but we weren't very good. Of course, it didn't matter to me that we weren't good as long as I got a chance to play. I enjoyed playing basketball, but football was my first love, and I still had my dream of becoming a great football player. Finally, I decided working at K-Bobs was not my life's ambition, so my new plan was to get myself in football shape, try to get accepted into Texas Southern University, and try to walk on to their football team.

The next few months consisted of me working out and eating lots of protein in an effort to gain some weight. I only weighed about 155 pounds, and I thought it was too small to compete at the collegiate level. I eventually got up to 175 pounds, and I didn't lose any speed in the process. My niece was my quarterback, and she would throw passes to me. She wasn't the best quarterback, so I would have her throw the ball as far as she could, and I would have to run as fast as I could to catch it. I enjoyed working out with the purpose of getting back on the field, putting those pads on again, and being part of a team would've been a dream come true.

My daily routine of going to work and working out went on for a few months, until I received a phone call about a potential job opportunity as a draftsman. It was decision time. I wanted to play football more than anything. Even though I was working, my parents were still supporting me since I was still living with them, eating their food, and using their electricity. If I were to go back to school, my parents would have been my main financial support system. If I were to take this job, I could make enough money to support myself. It was clear my parents were getting up in age, and they had already raised their eight children. I believe my parents would've supported me going back to school, but I thought it would be better for me to take the drafting job and start supporting myself. My parents had done so much for me I didn't feel I should put them in that position.

I didn't think about it at the time, but that decision was the official end of my dream of becoming a pro football player.

The job was in Grapevine, Texas, and it wasn't very far from Fort Worth, Texas, where my sister Jill lived. I moved in with her and her family until I was able to get my own place. It was a big culture shock for me after living in Jefferson most of my life and going to school at Kilgore, a relatively small town, and moving to Fort Worth, a metropolis. Getting used to the traffic was the biggest hurdle, but once again, I was able to adapt to my surroundings.

When I started my new job, it was a separate culture shock. Although the school system where I attended was integrated racially, most people in Jefferson lived extremely segregated lives. Even at Kilgore, I had more exposure to the white race, but most of my social experiences were segregated. My new job was with a very small company, about twenty employees, and I was the only African American. Everyone in authority at the company was white, and there were a few people of Latin decent working in the shop. My dealings with either of these ethnic groups were at best limited, but my family environment was such that I knew how to conduct myself in most situations, regardless of the racial makeup of the group. After a short while, it was as if I was meant to be in that environment. I've been the only African American at every job I've had since then.

There was a slight learning curve adapting the concepts in school with the company's way of doing things. I was the only draftsman on staff supporting four engineers, but I became very efficient at my job. These were the days when drafting was done on a drafting board with a pencil and a straight edge. My brother Joc was the first draftsman in our family, and he described this type of work as "taking candy from a baby." I had worked for this company almost two years when my bosses decided we should automate our drafting system. Computer-aided drafting or CAD had been around for a few years, but I had no knowledge of the concept. My bosses had such confidence in my ability, they allowed me to purchase all the company's CAD equipment and software. Being the only African American in the company and having the authority to make decisions of this magnitude really gave me a since of accomplishment, of which I'd never experienced.

Most people who use CAD software would take specialized courses or have a mentor of some sort to teach them the dynamics of the software. When I started using the software, I knew nothing about a computer, or how to draw with a computer. When I started, I spent most of the day drawing on the board because that's what I knew, then I would spend the rest of the day learning the software. Slowly, I would integrate the CAD drawings into my daily routine, and before you knew, it I was doing all the company drawings on the computer. It was a major accomplishment for me, both for that position and for any future opportunities.

My life was going great! I was establishing a career in a great city, making a decent living, and I was only about twenty-two years old, so I felt I had accomplished quite a bit for my age. Meanwhile, diabetes care had begun to grow by leaps and bounds; however, I was still in the dark ages in my personal care. I would get blood work done about every two months, while they were developing a means to test blood sugar on a daily basis. I did the best I could with the information I had, and I was still working out and playing all kinds of sports, like anyone who wasn't a diabetic.

There was a park near my office, where many people would play basketball, and when I discovered it, that's where I spent most of my leisure time. I made many connections at the park, where I learned about the various city basketball leagues going on in Grapevine. Though basketball wasn't my main sport, because I will forever be a football guy, I really enjoyed the time I was spending playing at the park and playing games in the leagues I was associated with.

The only thing missing from my life was a partner. I remember my mother coming up to visit one time, and we went to the grocery store to get things for her to cook dinner. We got separated in the store, but I found her in one of the aisles, and looking at her from a distance caused my mind to go to a bit of a melancholy state. On one hand, I was so grateful for my mother, who would come to visit me and cook me dinner; but on the other hand, how I longed for that special woman in my life, who would care for me the way my mother did. I was only twenty-two years old, but I thought time was wasting. And I needed my soulmate. Dinner was superb that night. My mother was a sensational cook. She spent the night, got up the next morning, and went back to Jefferson.

Soon after my mother's visit, I found an apartment and moved out of my sister's house. Getting my own apartment was a milestone that allowed me to be more independent and grow as an adult. I got all kinds of odd pieces of furniture that were given to me by friends and family. Needless to say, it was randomly put together. I never paid rent while living with my sister, so that new expense was something I had to get used to. The apartment was much closer to my job than my sister's house, and it cut down on my travel expense.

A few weeks later, I was shopping at a local mall, and when I'm out, I'm always aware of any females in my vicinity. I noticed a young lady walking in the mall alone, and from a distance, I thought she was quite attractive. After a while, I summoned up enough nerve to approach her. She seemed like a very nice lady. We talked for a while and exchanged numbers. Within a matter of weeks, she was dropping me off at work and taking my car to do whatever she had to do during the day. Part of me said it's not a good idea to let someone use your car when you've only known them for a few weeks. My family would've told me I was crazy if they knew, so I made a point of not revealing this information to my family.

At this point in my life, my hormones were raging. I wanted a life partner, but I really wanted a sexual relationship. This woman told me she was abstaining from any kind of sexual relationship, until she got married. I was accepting of her terms for a relationship; however, things were moving quickly. One day, she had my car, and she told me she was going to do my laundry. Thinking this was a potential mate taking care of my needs, I agreed to her offer. I thought she was going to wash and dry my clothes and fold them. Instead, she took all of my cloths to the dry cleaners and told me she needed money to get them out of the cleaners. This was my first red flag that our relationship was a bad idea. Somehow, I felt like when we were getting to know each other, I was having an out-of-body experience. I was clearly making very irrational decisions. I didn't know her that well. Sometimes, I thought she might steel my car when I let her use it during the day.

We had known each other about a month before she had moved in with me. I felt very uncomfortable with our living situation, but I allowed it to happen. I was so naive about the ways of the world, and she had an extremely forceful personality. She brought no assets to the relationship. She had no car or job. She didn't have any money. My life was unraveling right before my eyes because of this person. I didn't want my family to find out about her living with me, so after a few days, I went to her and said, "You're going to have to leave and find another place to live."

She came back to me and said, "I'm not leaving."

Making another irrational decision, I responded by saying, "If you won't leave, then, I guess we will have to get married."

I was hoping she would have the rational thought process to save me from myself and say there's no way we could get married, but instead, she agreed to the marriage. She seemed extremely happy, and we went around town telling everyone about our upcoming nuptials. Her family was very happy for us, but my family had never met her and was very concerned about my decision. My oldest brother, Joc, thought she had to be pregnant for us to decide to get married so quickly. Once again, I felt like I was having an out-of-body experience. I was watching myself making these terrible decisions, as if I were watching a TV movie. I felt as if I had no control of the situation.

One day, I was sitting at work with my head in my hands, thinking there's no way I can marry this woman, whom I barely knew, but something was compelling me to go through with the marriage. We managed to express our love for each other, even though I had no idea what it meant to love someone unconditionally. I think I made a conscious decision to tolerate her for the rest of our lives. I suppose if I had a better attitude, I could've loved her. For a couple of weeks more, we went through all the motions, and one random day, we decided today is the day. We got our marriage license, and that evening, her stepfather asked a neighbor of his, who was a minister, to come over to his house and perform the ceremony. The only people in attendance were myself, my soon-to-be wife, her mother, her step-father, her sister, and the minister.

Later that evening, we went to my sister's house to tell her the news, and while at her house, I called all of my family members to give them the news. I can only imagine the shock all of my family was feeling as I gave them the news about my marriage. Most of my family had not met my new wife, but we had our family reunion coming up in less than two months, so everyone was looking forward to finally meeting her. I knew the marriage was a mistake, but I didn't want to give the impression to my family that I didn't know what I was doing. I would put on the facade of a man, who truly loved his wife and was comfortable in my marital relationship.

When we got to the reunion, I was extremely nervous about my family meeting my new wife. My mother was a very sweet lady and nice to everyone she ever met. When they met, it seemed like they would grow to have a great relationship. Everyone else thought she was very pretty and that I had made a good choice on the surface. We made it through the weekend without any incidents. As time went on, you could start to feel the tension growing between my family and my wife. In some unconscious way, I may have allowed it to happen.

For all intents and purposes, we achieved the American dream as a couple. We purchased a house, bought several cars, and it seemed as if everything was falling into place like everything usually did in my life. The only thing I didn't anticipate was the fact that I now shared my life with another person who didn't share the same life experiences I had. I slowly learned things about my wife, and her adolescence, that I could've never imagined for myself, or anyone for that matter. She barely knew her biological father because he died while she was a very young child. Her stepfather wasn't very nurturing to her, or any of her two siblings from her mother's first marriage.

She left her mother's home at the age of sixteen, while I was barely removed from my parents' house, when we got married. Needless to say, she and I grew up in vastly different environments. She also dealt with many mental issues. I was not equipped to deal with any of the issues she had to live with, and overall, it could have been one of the reasons our marriage didn't last, although there were a plethora of reasons. We couldn't agree on much of anything. Many of our discussions would end with me coming over to her way of thinking. I'm almost ashamed to say, but sometimes, I would come over to her way of thinking. So if things didn't work out, I would be able to blame her. I'm no expert in marriage, but I do know it's not kind to deliberately set your partner up for failure.

There was one time, during our marriage, when we purchased a car based on her having a job and making the monthly payment every month. We argued for about a week. Her position was she needed a car to handle all the things she was involved with, including going to work every day, while my position wasn't very supportive at all. I would tell her she would quit the job, as she had done many times before, and I would be stuck with the monthly payment of which I felt I couldn't afford. We eventually purchased the car, and she had quit her job before the first payment was due. There I was paying every bill we had, and a new car payment on top of that. Even though I allowed my wife to make that decision, I had to live with the decision.

This was our marriage in a nutshell—two people diametrically opposed in every way, trying to come together to make a life. Eventually, I would grow to resent everything about my wife. We coexisted for several years. We were married for six years before my son, Sean Junior, was born. He was a beautiful baby, and I was so proud to be his father. I wanted to be the best father I could be for my son. The only example I had was my own father, who was the epitome of a stable provider. My father worked all the time, so he didn't have time to watch me play sports or be involved in anything that was going on in my life. I didn't resent my father for his lack of participation in my life because I think he did what he felt was important. The constant with humans is the propensity to make mistakes, and fortunately, there are times when we can learn from them and change. While I don't consider the way my father raised us as a mistake, more than I consider it a sign of those times I felt I could be more as a father. My ambition was to provide for my son and be involved in every aspect of his life. I realized he needed so much more than this, but if I could provide these things, he would be better off than many kids.

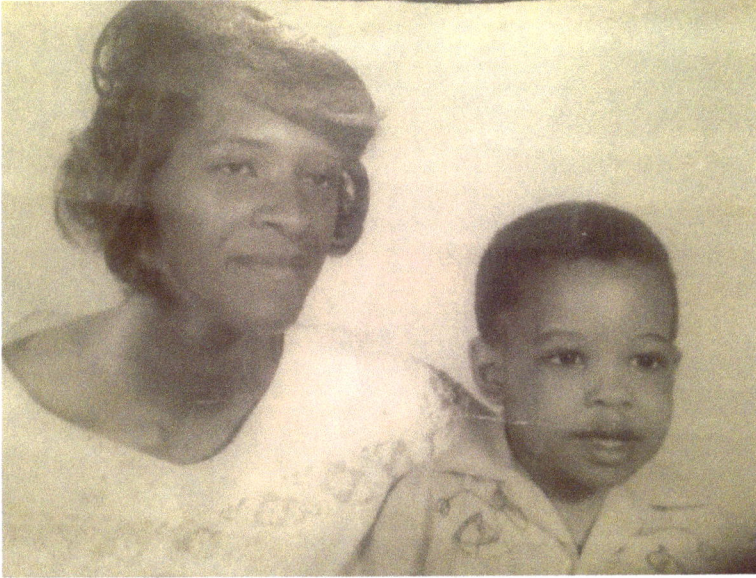

The oldest of eight siblings with me the youngest.

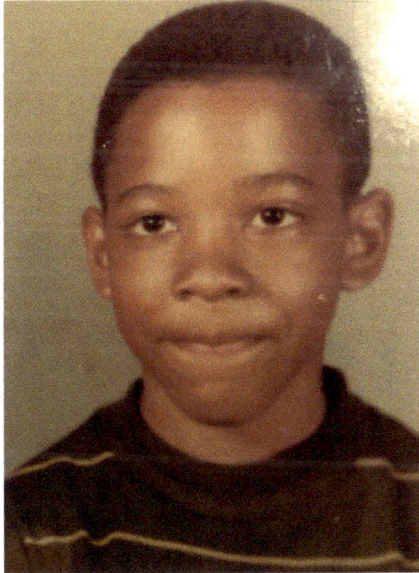

A young boy without a care
in the world only a plethora
of dreams not yet fulfilled.

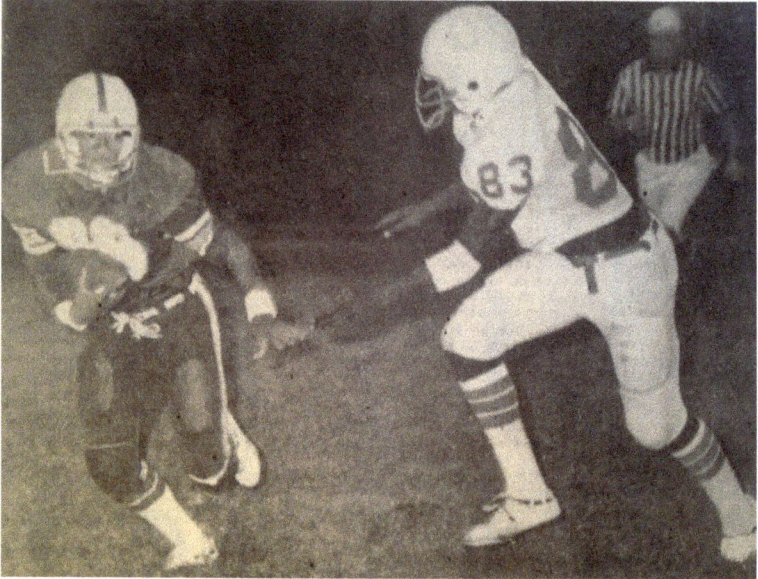

I was much smaller than many of my competitors
but my size was never a concern.

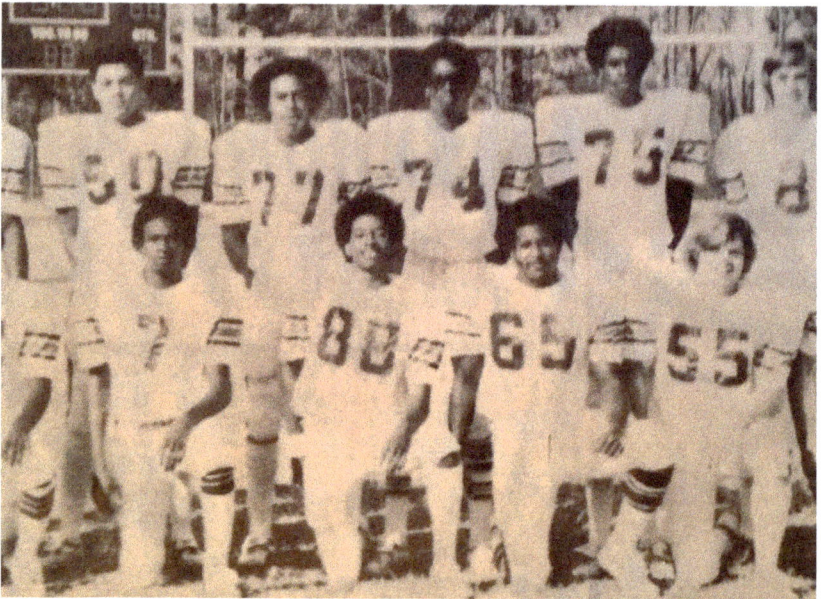

I loved everything about football. I loved being with my teammates, the
character building and the uniforms. I felt like a gladiator in the uniform.

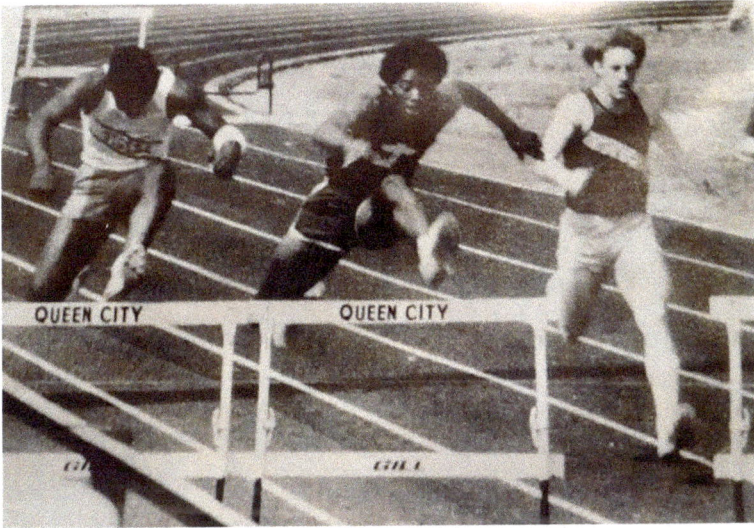

Throughout my junior high and high school years I was always able to compete in track and field despite my diabetes.

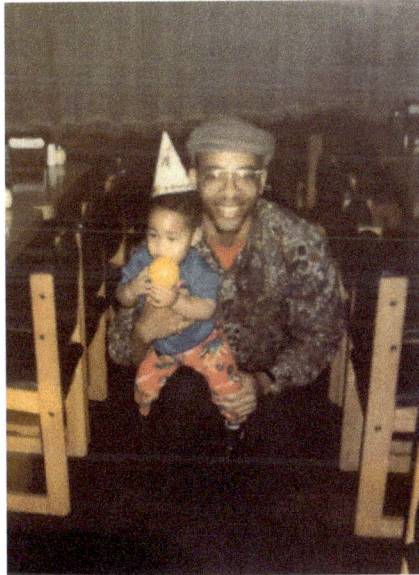

Sean, Jr. and I were at his first birthday party. He was just learning to walk and I was so proud.

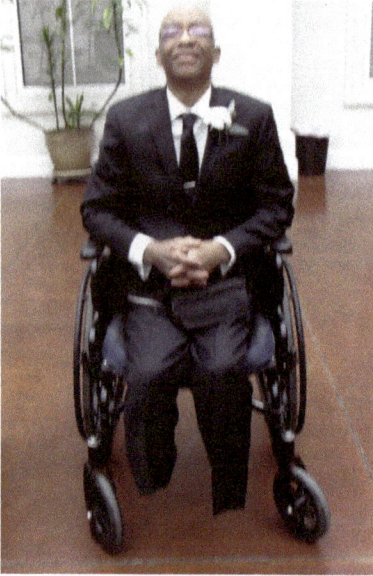

Even as an amputee I consider myself a fashionesta.

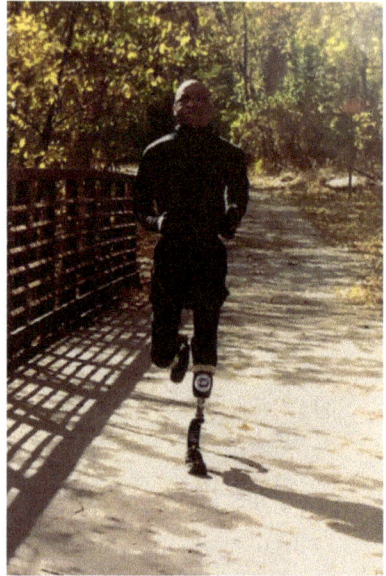

The first time I ran with my prosthetics I felt so free and alive with the wind in my face.

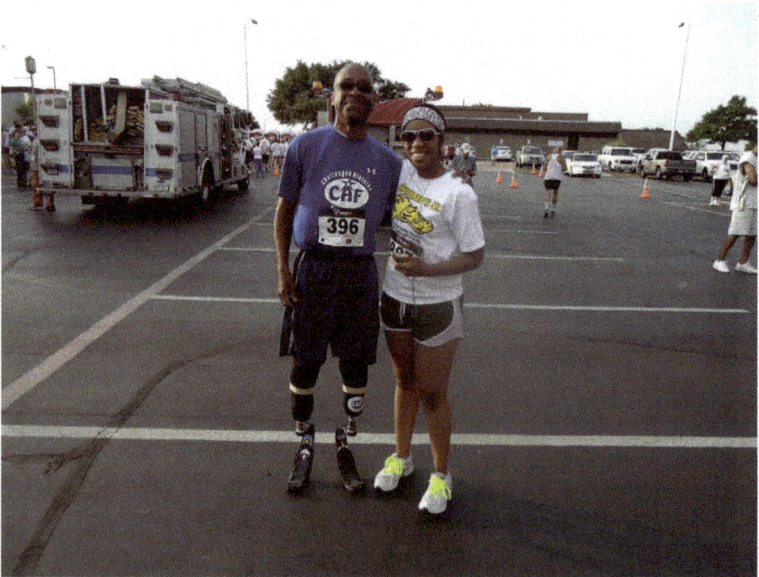

My niece Morgan and I are getting ready to run in a 5k race together.

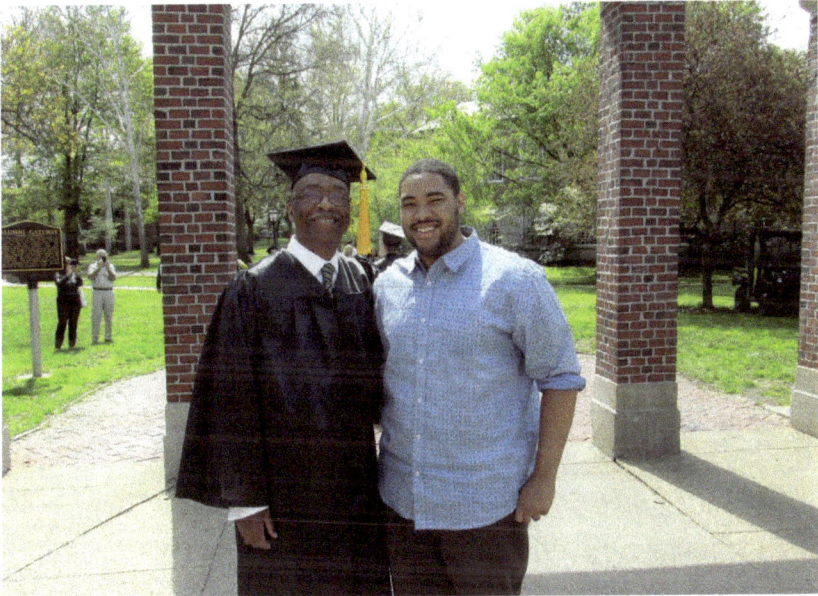

Sean, Jr. and I were in Athens, Ohio for my
graduation from Ohio University.

From my perspective, we struggled as a family just to make ends meet. We had to make decisions each month, regarding what bills would get paid in the household and what bills would not. I was making about forty thousand dollars a year, so I thought I was doing good. But with a wife whom I didn't communicate with on anything of importance, including financial issues, it seemed like we were on a poverty level. I could've made one hundred thousand dollars a year, and it still would not have been enough. We tried having bank accounts together, and it would always end in disaster. We could never balance a checkbook together. One account was in the negative so much the bank just decided to cancel the account. I had never been in a situation like that before, and it gave me another reason to resent my wife.

One day, my boss called everyone into the shop to explain how he had not taken a salary in about a year. The company was in major financial turmoil, and his first option was to cut everyone's salary by 25 percent. The next step would be to start laying off employees. I was already struggling financially, and hearing this news sent me directly into panic mode. I immediately started to look for another job to make up the 25 percent I was losing at my present position.

After about seven months of diligent searching for a new job, I found a job at Romeo Engineering. It didn't quite make up the 25 percent I lost, but I was so eager to make a change I jumped at the new opportunity. Romeo's main business was the manufacture of water jet-cutting machines. I had never heard of a water jet-cutting machine. I performed some of the same duties as in my previous job, but I was also allowed to become a programmer and a project manager. It was looking as if my career was moving in an upward direction, but financially, I was in the same depressing state.

We continued to go through a series of extraordinarily bad financial decisions. Finally, we decided to file for bankruptcy. It was another decision I was opposed to, but once again, I wanted to be able to blame my wife and not have any accountability. Ultimately, it reflected on our credit report as a couple, but all I saw was how this woman was dragging me down. After the bankruptcy, we fell behind on our mortgage payments, and one day, we just decided to abandon the house until it went into foreclosure. This was another extremely bad decision by a couple who had no clue of how to handle any situation.

I called this period in our lives as the vagabond stage. We moved a total of eleven times after we gave up the house. My mom and I talked about this years later, and she told me if we had come to her with this information, she would've helped us keep the house. I came to the conclusion that you can be vulnerable and tell others what's going on in your life, and I don't have to give the impression I have everything together.

Through all the process of changing jobs and the financial issues, I was still finding basketball leagues and running in races all over town. I played on a basketball team with a group of guys I knew from before I got married. We all played in a six-foot-and-under league. Before we started this team, I didn't know these gentlemen on a personal level. Our only relationship was basketball. As we played together and got to know each other on a more personal level, I learned how most of them were extremely unfaithful to their wives. We would sit around after games, and they would brag about some of their exploits with other women. At first, I couldn't believe how insensitive they were toward their wives. There was a time when I believed my personality was such that my environment would not influence my actions.

Looking at these men on my team, who seemingly have great lives while having extramarital affairs, made me question my fidelity to my wife. My wife and I didn't communicate; we didn't get along. She's dragging me down. We didn't agree on anything. God wants me to be happy. God would understand why I would cheat on my wife. I came up with many reasons why it would be beneficial for me to cheat on my wife. My happiness became the most important part of my life, while I neglected to see the importance of my wife's happiness. I was so out of touch with my wife's needs that it didn't matter if my infidelity would hurt her. In fact, I was so out of touch I didn't realize she had already been unfaithful to me in our marriage.

When I found out about her infidelity, my thought process was to hold it as another mark against her. This woman was a thorn in my side, plus, she had the nerve to cheat on me. I thought I had every right to cheat on her. Eventually, I got involved with a few different women during my marriage, and at the time, it seemed exciting. It was also exasperating the way I had to sneak around. All the time, I tried to put on the persona of a model citizen, a good husband, and father for the world, but deep down, I knew it wasn't true. My resentment of my wife grew into hate. Sometimes, when she would leave home, I would pray she would meet someone and just run away from home. Of course, that never happened. She would always find her way back home.

I'm reminded of a scripture, perhaps a bit late, when I think of this period in my life. In Ephesians 5:25, Paul tells husbands to love your wives just as Christ loved the church and gave himself up for her to make her holy, cleansing her by the washing with water through the word, and to present her to himself as a radiant church, without stain or wrinkle, or any other blemish but holy and blameless. In retrospect, I realize how I was so unloving to my wife and how she was seeking love but couldn't get it from her husband, who was pre-ordained to provide the love she needed. I was so ashamed of who I was back then, but praise God for his mercy and how he's taught me these things and allowed me to grow.

Life progressed with my wife and me. My time of competing in basketball leagues, three-on-three tournaments, flag football leagues, and five- and ten-kilometer races soon transitioned into getting my son involved in athletics. Sean Junior was bigger than most of the kids his age, so I would impress upon him a sense of athletic achievement throughout his adolescence. His first opportunity to play team sports was with the Diamondbacks, a tee-ball team. This began a long tradition of Sean Junior and I getting involved in all kinds of sports together.

In his younger athletic years, Sean Junior was just like most kids his age. He was just learning how to catch a ball with his glove and learning how to hit a baseball. It's heartwarming to see your offspring learn and grow at such an early age. You tend to project five and ten years down the road to what they can possibly become, almost never thinking they could go in a different direction than the one you've envisioned for them. He continued to play tee-ball, and he played basketball that year as well. The next year, I coached him in Coach Pitch baseball. I had never played on a baseball team in my life, so my knowledge of the game was limited at best. Although I didn't have a clue about coaching baseball, I wanted to at least give Sean Junior the experience of being part of a team. We won a few games, and we lost a few, but I think all the kids enjoyed the experience. And so did I.

It wasn't until the next year that Sean Junior started to come into his own as a baseball player. I didn't coach, so I wasn't able to hamper his progress. He was still eligible to play coach pitch that year, so he was assigned to a team called the Cardinals, coached by Coach Joe. Coach Joe was extremely knowledgeable about the game, and he knew how to teach the kids that age. He put Sean at catcher on defense. On most of the teams in that league, the catcher didn't do much, except retrieve the ball after the coach pitched it then threw it back to the coach, or at least, that was my understanding of the catcher position.

Coach Joe had developed Sean Junior into a viable part of the defense. They threw several kids out on the opposing teams at home plate due to Sean Junior's play. Whenever a kid would pop up near home plate, Sean Junior would be there to make the play. I remember one play in particular when a kid hit a piece of the ball, but the ball continued to go back toward the backstop. Most catchers at any age wouldn't have made that play because the ball is moving too fast, but Sean Junior made the play on the ball and got the batter out. The crowed was amazed at the ability of this young boy, and I was an extremely proud father.

Sean Junior's offensive ability was equally, if not more, impressive. The other coaches in the league would cringe every time Sean Junior came up to bat. He would typically hit a home run because, even though he didn't hit the ball over the fence, most of the outfields of the other teams weren't able to gather the ball before he was able to run all of the bases. Sean Junior and his team achieved a great deal of success in the two years he played with Coach Joe and the Cardinals, and I attribute most of their success to the coaching Coach Joe provided to the kids.

Football was my game, so when Sean Junior started to play football, I was able to give him insight based on my knowledge of the game. His first little league team was the Hallmark Eagles. It was a bit of a culture shock for both of us because everyone on the team was African American. When Sean Junior played baseball with the Cardinals, he was the only African American on the team. I thought it would be a good experience for him to be involved with people of his own race. The kids on this team did seem to be a bit more aggressive than the white kids he played baseball with. Most of that can probably be attributed to the socioeconomic conditions African Americans find themselves in. At the age of seven, Sean Junior didn't quite grasp the difference in culture, and he got along well with all the kids on both teams.

Like I said before, Sean Junior was a big kid for his age, so in this league, kids who weighed over a certain amount couldn't play positions where they could run the ball—running back, quarterback, etc. Unfortunately Sean Junior exceeded this weight limit, and he was relegated to play offensive and defensive lineman. I think Sean Junior was more interested in *Ninja Turtles* and things of that nature more than football. He did continue to play that year, and he did quite well, but his interest was limited. He played mostly because I wanted him to follow my legacy, than of his own volition.

The next season, Sean Junior played in a different league in Haltom City, and he played with the Buffalos. Once again, Sean Junior was playing on the offensive and defensive line. When I played, I always played skilled positions, like quarterback or wide receiver, so I couldn't give him the best teaching on how to play his positions. With the help of his coaches and Sean Junior's willingness to learn, he became a very good offensive and defensive lineman.

Sean Junior continued to play different sports. Mostly football and baseball, but he did have opportunities to play some basketball during his childhood. As a family, we moved around on a regular basis. We moved a total of ten times between 1997 and 2008. Our home was foreclosed in 1996, and it was just one bad financial decision after the other. Physically, I thought I was doing well with my diabetes, but I could've been doing much better. Checking blood sugar daily was still a foreign concept to me. I knew how important insulin was to my survival, but I didn't understand how to regulate it according to my blood sugar. My relationship with my wife wasn't good because I blamed her for our financial situation. Needless to say, life was difficult for our entire family.

During one of our moves, I had just about had it with my marriage, when a gentleman by the name of JJ knocked on our door to invite us to church. It was at a time when I was actively seeking some spiritual guidance. He was a part of the International Church of Christ. I was familiar with the Church of Christ, but I had never heard of this particular group. My wife and I decided to visit the church one Sunday. I noticed several things about the church. The first was they didn't have a designated building. This introduced to me, for the first time in my life, the concept of church being within the heart and not a building. The second thing I noticed was that everyone greeted each other with hugs. Growing up, my family wasn't a touchy-feely group, and personal space was cherished, so it took me off guard.

The one thing that really caught my attention about the church was that so many races and ethnic backgrounds were represented. My church experience had been all churches contained members of the same race. In all Christian churches we're taught how God loves everyone, regardless of race, creed, or color, but I never questioned why people of different races didn't worship together. This was something that intrigued me and, eventually, drew me in. We met some interesting people who asked my wife and I to study the Bible. I was a consistent reader of the Bible, but like the Ethiopian eunuch, I never had a true understanding of the Bible. I understood who Jesus was and how he was crucified and rose from the dead, but I didn't understand how the whole Bible related to that sequence of events and how it would affect my life.

My wife and I agreed to study the Bible with the church. When we studied, they separated my wife and me. She studied with a group of women, and I studied with a group of men. The church had developed a series of study that I felt gave you some practical knowledge about the Bible, Jesus, who we are as human beings, and what our purpose is on this earth. The men I studied with were all of European descent, but it really didn't bother me. When we started the studies, each man would share about their lives and how they became Christians. Something else I noticed about the church was they didn't use the term *Christian*. Their philosophy was the term *Christian* is only used twice in the Bible, but the term *disciple* is used many times in the Bible to describe Jesus's followers. They identified themselves as disciples rather than Christians.

These men I studied with were extremely vulnerable with me, and they shared things about their lives that, personally, I would've never shared at the time. These were things you hear about on the news. The things they shared were so explicit in nature, but they explained to me how when we share these things, it allows us to hold each other accountable for the sin in our lives. I noticed the close bond between the men in that study, by the way they shared the most intimate details of their lives. I had friends in school and teammates on various teams I was a part of, but close relationships like this, I had never known.

They called the first study the Word study. The importance of this study was for the person in the study to make a firm commitment to read the Bible on a daily basis. I had no problem making a commitment to read the Bible daily because I was reading the Bible consistently before the study. The scriptures used in the study gave me reasons why I should be reading daily. Before that study, I just thought reading the Bible was the right thing to do.

The next study was called the discipleship study. This is where they taught me their views about the term *disciple*, as opposed to the term Christian. They believed the term *Christian* was used in the Bible more as a derogatory representation of Jesus's followers, but the term *disciple* was more of a representation of honor and prestige. In all my years of reading the Bible, I had never questioned these words and how they were used in the context of faith in God, but it did open my eyes to a deeper level of understanding.

The studies gave me an incredible insight into the Bible, and many things I had read in the past, but never truly understood. I also developed some great friendships with the men I was studying with. I had relationships with men prior to my time of study, but never before had I grown to know men on a heart level, as we started to refine our relationships. In retrospect, I suppose these men could have been putting on some sort of act to draw me into the church, but I don't know, and neither did I ever believe that was the case. I believe these men were genuine in their concern for my spiritual well-being.

The next time we got together to study, we talked about sin. Their philosophy on sin was that no sin was greater than another sin, but all sins separate us from God. And all sins can be forgiven through Jesus Christ. I had an understanding about Jesus's death on the cross and how he did this for the sin of the world, but this study made Jesus's death more personal to me than I had ever envisioned it before. Each man in the study with me shared about his personal sin during the study. On one hand, I was amazed at how these men could share such intimate details about their lives, things most people wouldn't dare tell a soul. On the other hand, I knew this was an attempt to get me to share the sin in my life for which I was extremely reluctant to share.

It was a very uncomfortable study for me because there was some sin in my life I was so ashamed of I had never really mentioned it in prayer, while alone with just God and me. By this time, the relationships we had forged during the time of our studies would allow me to share some of my darkest secrets. Up to this point in my life, people considered me the model citizen. My sinful nature was not inclined to give any other impression. I wanted to be the man I portrayed on the outside, and I trusted these men enough to share my sin.

I told the men in the study about my infidelity with other women during my marriage. Confessions like mine were not uncommon in studies of this nature, as I would later find out when I started to study the Bible with other men. I was ashamed of my sin, but I didn't feel any judgment toward me. All I felt was support and understanding. The next study was the Cross. We talked about what my sin does to me and the people in my life, but also what it did to Jesus and why he endured such an excruciating death for me. All these studies gave me a greater appreciation for Jesus Christ and his sacrifice. We read scripture that I had read before, but most of it, I never comprehended. After studying with these men, Jesus's death had a profound effect on my life.

At the same time I was studying the Bible, my wife was studying with the women. When we would talk, I could, since she was going through some of the same emotions I was going through. We were never honest with each other about our sin, but after the studies, we were able to confess the truth about our marriage. We decided to forgive each other and move forward. Many times during the studies, we talked about a triangular relationship between man, his wife, and God. The idea is as you and your wife grow closer to God, you, in turn, grow closer to each other. This concept was evident in our relationship in the weeks and months to follow.

My wife and I decided to be baptized and join the church. Both of us had been baptized before, but during the studies, we gained a new understanding of baptism and its significance. We planned to get baptized at an upcoming service the church was having at the Dallas Convention Center. It was a huge service with thousands of people in attendance. The pastor of our church baptized me, then I got out of the baptismal, and I proceeded to baptize my wife.

Both my wife and I became extremely active in the church. The church was very evangelistic, and it was because someone (JJ) invited us to church, and the fact that I felt an obligation to Jesus, we, in turn, began to evangelize. It was never my personality to go out and speak to strangers, but eventually, I got on board with inviting people to church, and even asking people to study the Bible. The image of the church seemed to be very benevolent and philanthropic, but they didn't seem to have many assets. We didn't own a building, so we rented a meeting place. I always assumed all churches owned their buildings, so this was another new thing I had to get used to. Many of the philanthropic efforts were funded by the members of the church or by the members hitting the streets, asking for donations. Many people were offended by our asking for donations, but I found many people who would donate to what they might consider to be a legitimate cause.

My wife and I began to call ourselves Disciples of Christ rather than Christians, just as everyone else in the church did. The term *disciple* was also used as a verb based on a scripture from Matthew 28:18–20, where before he ascends to heaven, Jesus tells his disciples to go and make disciples of all nations, baptizing them, and teaching them to obey everything he has commanded them. When new disciples were baptized, he or she would be given a discipleship partner, who would help them with all aspects of following Christ. We studied the Bible with many people, and "discipled" many couples. It was a powerful and impactful period in my life. My wife and I were growing in our relationship with God and each other.

TRANSPLANT

The relationships I had built with men in the church were unlike any I had in my life with other men. One of my most meaningful discipleship partners was with a gentleman named Mike. Most of my relationships before the church were with African American men, but Mike was white. He knew all the intimate details about my life, and I knew everything about his life. We always talked about the sin in our lives and held each other accountable for our sin. We would pray together constantly. There's something about praying together that brings people closer together. We would go out to meet people, invite them to church and to study the Bible. We did all this because we felt it was our purpose in life.

Mike and I studied the Bible with several men, and we eventually baptized a few of them. There was no inconvenient time for us to plan a study. Sometimes, we would get together before work or late in the evenings to help someone have a relationship with Jesus Christ. We were living out our purpose of seeking and saving the lost. Men would see our relationship and would want the same thing in their lives. We really made a difference in the city we lived in.

My life as a disciple was tremendous. My purpose was clear, but diabetes had begun to take a toll. For the first time since living with my parents, I was seeing a doctor on a regular basis. I started getting lots of swelling in my ankles, which was a sure sign of something going wrong. My blood pressure was extremely out of control, and the doctor put me on medication for my blood pressure. Before this, I was only taking insulin, for which, I was very proud of the fact that I only took one medication with my illness. I wasn't working out as much as I did before this time, but I still had opportunities to work out.

Throughout my life, I always depended on my ability to work out to triumph over my disease. I thought that working out would get me through any physical ailment I could face. If I had high blood sugar, I would run a few miles to bring it down. Now, I had to depend on pills to regulate my blood pressure. Diligence in taking blood pressure medication helped my blood pressure a bit, but it didn't keep me from being cursed with renal failure. I knew practically nothing about renal failure; however, I learned quickly. The main lessons learned about this disease were that the only treatments were dialysis and that the only cure is kidney transplant.

A prerequisite for renal failure is typically diabetes or high blood pressure. I also learned that compared to Caucasians, the prevalence of renal failure is about 3.7 times greater among African Americans. These three facts increased my odds for developing kidney disease exponentially. Here I was, in the prime of my life, with a wife and a young son, and now, I have to deal with another disease. It was another obstacle in a long history of circumstances I had to deal with.

A couple of months passed, and I finally got to the point where my kidney function was so depleted I had to start dialysis. I didn't understand the process of dialysis, so I was embarking on a new frontier. I had surgery on my right arm to develop the injection sight used for dialysis, called a fistula. I was told the surgery went well, and I would be able to use the fistula within a few weeks. In the meantime, I had to get what is called Permacath to dialyze immediately and use it until my fistula matured enough to use. Typically, a Permacath is a temporary solution for dialysis because it is attached directly to the heart and is subject to infection.

The first day I went to the dialysis clinic, I was so nervous. I had never known anyone who had to go through dialysis, so the whole thing was a mystery. When I walked into the clinic, I noticed about forty patients sitting in reclining chairs, and each patient had a five-foot-tall machine next to them. Each patient had Poly-Flow tubing attached to them that ran through the machine. The tubing would also run through a huge filter called a dialyzer. I had seen this item before at work when my company was commissioned to build a machine used to test dialyzers for consumption. It was a serial moment because when my company was working on this machine, I had no idea what the item being tested would be used for. Never could I have imagined this item would be used to save my life.

The patient's blood runs through the tubing, through the dialyzer, and back to the patient—essentially performing the same task the kidney would perform. In the beginning, it's a frightening thought to see your blood running through this tubing, but after a while, you get used to it. I had to get used to it because this was my life for four hours, three times a week for the foreseeable future, and possibly forever. As I adjusted to the process, it became almost second nature to me. I continued to work during the day, and I would go to dialysis every Monday, Wednesday, and Friday evenings. I couldn't travel anymore for work because of my schedule, but I was able to work in the office. During dialysis, most patients watch television or sleep. Some would read, and others would bring computers and work on them.

The demographic of the patients at this dialysis center seemed quite common. Most of the patients were elderly African American, although there were a few white people and a few people of Latin descent. This did coincide with the information I had concerning the ethnicity of people on dialysis. I considered myself relatively young compared to most of the patients at the clinic. It was difficult to see myself in this situation, but I still had a positive outlook on life.

As weeks went by, my medical team discovered my fistula wasn't going to mature enough to use for dialysis. We had to go through another surgery to fix the fistula, so we could use it. Again, they said the surgery went well, and I should be able to use the fistula in a few weeks. I was still using the Permacath for dialysis, and I continued to use it for another four months. The fistula never matured to the point where I was able to use it during dialysis. The next option was to put a graph in my left arm. A fistula is created when a vein and an artery are tied together to form a loop for the dialysis process. A graph is created by inserting a synthetic tube between the vein and artery to make the loop necessary for dialysis.

During all the surgeries, and about six months of dialysis, I was going through the process of getting on the transplant list. I had to go through many test to get approved to be on the list. It took about four months for me to be approved for the list, and I was put on the list to receive a kidney/pancreas transplant. This would both take me out of renal failure and essentially cure my diabetes. Before I started this process, I knew nothing about a pancreas transplant, but I thought it would be great to cure both diseases at one time.

Finally, the surgery was set up for my graph to be placed in my left arm. Once again, I was told the surgery went well, and in a few weeks, I would be able to use it for dialysis. Approximately one week after the graph surgery, I received a call from the transplant coordinator to let me know there may be a possible kidney/pancreas available for transplant. They called me late Sunday night, so I had to be at the hospital early Monday morning to go through the testing to see if the organs were compatible.

The hospital completed its test for compatibility, and before I knew it, I was being prepped for the surgery. Never before had I been through a surgery of this magnitude, so my main concern was coming out of the surgery alive. My wife called all my friends from church and my family, so everyone was praying for a successful surgery and a quick recovery. The focus of my prayer during this time was extremely selfish, to say the least. It's difficult to pray for the plight of children in third-world countries when you are going through a situation like this.

The surgery took about four hours to complete, and I woke up late on that evening of March 4, 2004, in the recovery room with a new kidney and pancreas. I did wake up, so that meant I survived the surgery. I was lying there in much pain and praying to God that He would deliver me from the pain. It was so excruciating I didn't know if I was going to make it back to a normal life. The only control I had over my circumstances was my ability to pray. Every moment spent awake for the next day or two was devoted to prayer.

The next few days were difficult. I was still in a lot of pain, and I had a tube running to my stomach through my nose. Immediately, I had to start taking the immune suppressant drugs to fight rejection of the new organs. I barely could swallow the medication with this tube running through my throat. They finally removed the tube running to my stomach, which was a major milestone in my recovery. I was able to swallow the medication better, and I was able to start a somewhat normal diet consisting of Jell-O and chicken broth. Soon, I could eat and drink anything I wanted. In renal failure, you are on fluid restriction because your kidneys can't process the fluid. You don't realize how much you can take drinking for granted until you are on dialysis, and your fluids are restricted.

About two weeks after the surgery, I was able to go home. Leaving the hospital was quite surreal, knowing that I have a new lease on life. With the new kidney, I no longer had to go to dialysis, and with this new pancreas, I am no longer a diabetic. The implications of no more diabetes after living most of my life as a diabetic were astounding. No more insulin injections, and more freedom with my diet were the biggest changes I was looking forward to. It was beyond my imagination to think that one day I would be free of all of my afflictions.

The support received from family, people from church, and even my coworkers was amazing. Everyday members at our church would make dinner for me and my family. We were also having some car issues at the time of the transplant, so one church member allowed us to use their really nice car for about three weeks after the surgery. I wasn't working at this time, and we had a very substantial electric bill that was coming due. Our church took up a collection to pay that bill for us. I didn't work for about six weeks after the surgery, but my boss was extremely considerate enough to keep my job open until I was ready to come back. I worried about all these things, but it seemed that everywhere I looked, God was blessing my family.

A few weeks after my transplant, my transplant coordinator gave me some information about my donor. She was an eighteen-year-old white girl who was riding in the back of a pickup truck that was involved in an accident. I could never be labeled as a race activist, but I am aware of the strife between the races in America. To have such a life-saving gesture occur in my life from a white person would dispel any of my apprehension about race. Later on, there was an event, where me, along with several individuals who received organs from this young lady, were allowed to meet her family. It was an amazing experience to see so many people who would benefit from this young lady's kind gesture of organ donation. Everyone showed their great appreciation to her family, and after such a devastating loss, the family was inspired to see their daughter live on through all the organ recipients.

MIDDLE FINGER

My first experience with extremity pain and amputation was with my left index finger. I notice a spot underneath my fingernail and a slight pain, but didn't really give it much thought. That is, until one night, when my family was visiting my father in Jefferson when I was trying to sleep the pain became so excruciating that I couldn't sleep. As days passed, the pain got more severe. I started to see a vascular doctor who would determine that it was a vascular issue.

Vascular disease is common among diabetics, especially when they have enormous shifts in blood sugar levels. Before the invention of the glucose monitor, diabetics didn't have the luxury of monitoring blood sugar on a daily basis. It really came down to a guessing game of how you might feel as oppose to an accurate reading of your blood sugar. Unfortunately, I was never asymptomatic when it came to my blood sugar, unless it was extremely low, and I was having a reaction to the insulin.

My doctor didn't think my pain was diabetes related. Remember, I wasn't a diabetic at this point because of my kidney/pancreas transplant. The doctor determined it was a problem with a graph I received in my left arm for dialysis a few years before, in which I never used. I got my transplant one week after the graph was installed. His suggestion was to tie off the blood supply to the graph there by increasing blood flow, and that would take care of the problem with my finger.

The doctor performed the procedure to tie off the blood supply to the graph, but afterwards, I was still in pain. And the spot underneath my fingernail was growing even extending and onto the very tips of my finger. The pain was really aggravating at night, when I was trying to sleep. I would be up all night, walking in circles to alle-

76

viate the pain. Sleep deprivation began to affect my job performance, and I was running out of options on what to do about this problem.

Someone suggested I see a pain management doctor to help me. When I got there, he told me about the different procedures they could do to take away my pain, but at this point, I was a bit skeptical. After weeks of treatment with pain management, I was still in pain, but the spot had seemed to stop growing.

Finally, I went to see a plastic surgeon. She told me she could remove the spot by amputating a small portion of my finger, and hopefully, it would take away my pain. By this time, I had gone through so many months of agony that I was willing to try anything. It was a day surgery, and they released me immediately after the surgery. For about a week, I continued to have pain from the surgery, but after that, my finger was as good as new. My fingernail grew back, and you could hardly tell there was a problem. Little did I know this was the beginning of my relationship with amputations.

One day, I started to experience pain in my left middle finger, but there was no injury to the finger, similar to the situation I had with my index finger before. The pain just seemed to come from know where. Once again, I began to lose sleep because of the pain, and once again, it started to affect my job performance. Working as an engineer/project manager put a great deal of pressure on me to get projects out of the door to the customer site within a certain time frame. Between the pain I was experiencing and the anxiety I was feeling from my boss, if I didn't meet deadlines, put me in a position of making regretful decisions in all aspects of my life.

Slowly, I noticed my finger turning darker in color, and the pain increasing. It was different from the last episode with my index finger because it wasn't just the tip of the finger, but the whole finger. No one, including the doctors, had a clue of what was happening to me. Finally, the vascular doctor who thought I had an issue with the graph implanted in my left arm for dialysis discovered that my veins had so much calcification that my fingers on my left hand had very little blood flow.

My doctor suggested a procedure to remove a vein from my right leg and place it in my left arm to bypass the more calcified veins and, hopefully, save my finger. Based on my childhood experiences with doctors, I just assumed if you go to the doctor for a problem with your body, the doctor can fix it. I had to come to the realization that these people in the medical field weren't magicians, and they may not have all the answers.

We decided to go through with the bypass procedure. I was in so much pain I was willing to do anything to take it away. They started the procedure by making a long incision on my right inner thigh. The incision went from my groin to near my knee in order to remove the vein they would use in my left arm for the bypass. When the procedure was over, there was a very pronounced heartbeat along the inside of my upper left arm. I was also left with staples running along the incision on my right thigh. It looked like they had installed a zipper on my leg.

Both I and the doctors thought with the increased circulation to my hand, we would create a healing pattern. Things didn't go as planned. The pain continued, and the whole finger turned black. I began to notice a very distinct odor coming from my finger. I've never experienced the odor of a dead decaying body, but I knew the scent coming from my finger was the scent of death. I remember, one day, when I was going through this. Looking at my hand, I was trying to move my fingers. Every finger would move accept the middle finger. I thought, if I tried some sort of mental telepathy, I could force it to move, but I had no control. It was a dead appendage that permeated to the point that I knew the next step was the amputation of the finger.

The vascular doctor I was working with asked me right before my surgery if I wanted to lose the whole hand, or just the finger that was causing all the pain? I was extremely put off by his question, and I thought it was very insensitive of him to suggest taking my hand. Fortunately, my hand surgeon had the common sense to only concentrate on the finger.

By this time, surgery was a common part of my existence. Nevertheless, I was still very nervous about going under the knife again. I had a hand surgeon who was quite experienced, so he somewhat put me at ease.

After I came out of surgery, it was like a miracle. I had a huge bandage on my left hand, where my finger was, but there was virtually no pain. The surgeon came into my hospital room to change the bandage, and I was afraid to look at the wound. Finally, I took a peek at the wound, and it was as ugly as I thought, but the pain was gone. And I was happy. My only issue now was returning to my regular life without my left middle finger. I had concerns about how society would treat me more than how I would function without the finger.

When all the bandages were removed, and the healing process was complete, most people hardly noticed the area where the finger was amputated. As far as functionality was concerned, I could do everything I did before the amputation, so it really didn't affect my lifestyle in a significant way. When this happened, it reminded me of animals that loses a limb. If you see a dog with three legs, it doesn't have to go through extensive rehabilitation. It just goes on with its life.

STAND UP

After a few years of being in church, life was wonderful! My marriage was a great place. My wife and I had worked out our differences, and Sean Junior was very involved in the church. Overall, I was extremely happy about my life. One day, out of the blue, my wife accused me of having an affair. Trust can be quite fickle when it has been betrayed in the past. I thought our issues with infidelity had been conquered after we studied the Bible, but something triggered her feelings that I was cheating again. I tried as best I could to convince her that her feelings were unfounded, but she wouldn't listen.

We were on the brink of divorce before we studied the Bible. After studying the Bible, hope was renewed in me that our marriage could withstand anything. Unfortunately, studying the Bible didn't improve our communication skills. Throughout my life, up to that point, I had always been quite reserved in the way I communicated, while my wife was very boisterous when she would communicate with others. She would let you know how she felt, when she felt it, and she would take no prisoners if you know what I mean.

During this argument that came out of the blue, she asked me to leave our home, where I was paying the rent, so I left. I leaned on all the relationships I had built in the church for support, but my pride was so strong I didn't ask anyone for a place to stay. After driving around for a few hours, desperation for a place to stay set in. I had the idea to contact one of the women with whom I had an affair with in the past. I didn't know how to contact her since I had deleted all that information, but I did remember where she worked during our affair. I went by her place of employment and found out she no longer worked there. This was a blessing in disguise, as I would've reverted to my old sins.

I went to the Salvation Army to find a place to stay. They made me feel less than a person immediately, when I walked in the door. It was a cold winter day, and I was wearing a hat when I walked in the door. The first thing the gentleman said to me when I walked in was "Remove your hat when you come inside." I was expecting some semblance of compassion when I went there. This was the Salvation Army. I was so offended by his greeting without saying a word, I turned and walked out.

After exhausting all my options, I decided to sleep in my car and go to truck stops to shower. Our budget was tight as a family, and I still had to maintain the household that I was just kicked out of. Coming up with a $1.50 for a shower would have been a stretch. While sitting in my car, contemplating my dire situation, my wife called me and suggested I come back home. It hadn't been a full day since she told me to leave, but I was happy she had changed her mind. When I got home, she told me she didn't want me to share our bedroom. I had to explain the situation to Sean Junior on why I wasn't sleeping in my bed. I relied on a scripture during this period. In John 16:33, Jesus says "In this world you will have trouble, but take heart. I've overcome the world."

I wanted to conceal the issues I was having with my wife from my son, but he was growing up and becoming a man right before my eyes. I couldn't imagine going through something like this with my parents when I was that age, and I never imagined putting my own son through this.

Things never really got back to the way they were before these accusations, but we eventually started to sleep together. And we went on with our lives. My wife started to correspond with some people from the Seventh-day Adventist Church, and she began to live by some of the doctrine taught in their church. I was completely opposed to her desire to change her religious attitudes, but I was willing to support her decision to change churches. It wasn't enough for me to support her decision to change. She wanted Sean Junior and me to follow her in her decision.

In our church, we had a term for people who walked away from the church and didn't follow the Bible. When this happened, we said that person had "fallen away." In my mind, the church had saved my marriage, and I had an obligation to the church, to Jesus, and to God to remain faithful and continue my relationship with the church. I had witnessed people who had "fallen away." Couples who met in the church, and their marriages were based on biblical principles. These couples would leave the church and eventually break up. It was heartbreaking to see these couples fall apart after coming together with God as the main focus. In my mind, if we left the church, our marriage was doomed for failure.

The Seventh-day Adventist Church meets on Saturday, their Sabbath. I reluctantly went to that church with my wife on occasion, but sometimes, I would pretend to have to go to work, so I could get out of the semi-commitment I had made to my wife. We would argue about my working on the Sabbath, until one day, in the middle of an argument, she called me Satan. That label she had put on me marked the beginning of the end of our marriage. Her image of me resonated so profoundly I began in many ways to live up to her assessment.

We stayed together for couple of more years, but life was so different from the time we were faithful in our church. My prayer life had taken a major dive. It wasn't that I had stopped believing in God, but I did feel as if I had lost control of my life. We eventually stopped going to church altogether. I would spend more time at work, even though I wasn't working. It was an attempt to get away from my wife and the life we had stumbled into at home. Each day after work, I would come home and look at the front door and ask myself, *Do I really want to continue to subject myself to everything that goes on behind that door?* Until one day, when I decided not to go through that door ever again. From that day, I never lived with my wife again.

I never had a conversation with my wife about how I was feeling, or why I didn't want to be married any more. I just walked out without any explanation. Up to that point in my life, it was difficult to make decisions, but when I made that decision, it was written in stone. My son was out of high school, and I felt he was the main casualty in the whole thing. He continued to live with my wife, and

I think our separation changed my son's and my relationship for a time. He spent about a year not speaking to me after the break up.

After a while, I had started a new relationship with a woman I had met while working in Ohio. Her name was Theo. It was a beautiful relationship, even though we couldn't spend much time together because of the distance, but we managed to see each other monthly for about two years. Either she would come to Texas, or I would go to Ohio. She was the first woman in my life that I had an intimate connection with. There was a communication between us that I had never experienced before with anyone. We made plans to get married as soon as my first marriage was dissolved.

I moved in with my sister, Carlotta, and her family when I left my wife. They were very helpful to me at a time, when I couldn't do much for myself. During this time, I was in a great deal of pain in my lower extremities. The pain was so excruciating I would have to go to the hospital on occasion, so they could treat the pain. In the hospital, they would give me an IV pain medication called Deloted that would take the pain away for about fifteen minutes, and the pain would come back. I would have to wait two hours before I could take the medication again. I would always count the minutes until I could take the medication and get some relief. During this time, I was walking on crutches because the pain in my foot was so severe.

When I got out of the hospital, my sister and her daughter, Morgan, would continue to take me to doctor's appointments. One day, Carlotta took me to an appointment that would change my life dramatically. While we were in the doctor's office, he told me they would probably have to amputate my foot. At that moment, I was thinking, *If this will take away the pain, let's do it.* Later on, Carlotta mentioned when the doctor said "amputate," she almost fainted. It was almost ironic the different response we both had to the same news, but then, she couldn't fully understand the pain I was living with.

I left that appointment and went straight to the hospital, where they began to give me pain medication again. During all this talk about amputation, I found out that my transplanted kidney was failing, and I would have to start dialysis again. With so many negative things going on in my life, I felt like I was having some sort of out-of-body experience. I had gone through many trials in my life, but never could I have imagined what was happening to me. A few years earlier, I was playing city league basketball and running in races every weekend. It seemed like I was a lifetime and a different person removed from those days.

Soon, the orthopedic surgeon came to talk to me about the surgery. He said he will have to amputate my left leg just a few inches below my knee, and he would have to amputate half of my right foot. When my family heard this, they wanted me to get a second opinion, but I was in so much pain I was ready to get it done. On January 26, 2010, they did the surgery, and there I was with my left leg gone and part of my right foot gone. After the surgery, my doctor came to me and told me the circulation in my right leg wasn't sufficient, so they would need to perform the same amputation on my right leg. I was more reluctant to go through this surgery because I thought it would affect my ability to walk again. The doctor explained that if I didn't get this done soon, it could get worse, and they would have to amputate higher up my leg. On January 29, 2010, they amputated my right leg, just a few inches below my knee.

Immediately, the hospital started sending rehabilitation personnel to my room to teach me things, like how to transfer from the bed to a chair or how to transfer from a wheelchair to the toilet. An able-bodied person rarely thinks of these things and takes them for granted, but when it became a necessity to think of these things, I found it very difficult to accomplish. A couple of days after my amputations the hospital moved me to the rehab wing of the hospital. This is where I learned many things that would help me function as a bilateral below knee amputee. I worked with several physical therapist and occupational therapist, who gave me the tools necessary to get started.

One day, a physician whom I had never met before came to my room, and he gave me a bit of advice I've lived by since that day. He told me, "After all you've been through, you can still accomplish everything you were able to do in the past. You will just have to find a different way of accomplishing those things." That advice resonated with me as I modified my lifestyle. My sister's home wasn't exactly disability friendly, but each day, I learned how to achieve different task. I had a portable toilet, and my sister created a screen to make trips to the restroom more discrete. It was very embarrassing because my sister had to clean the toilet every time I used it. My next goal was to learn to go to the bathroom. This was no small task, considering my wheelchair couldn't fit through the bathroom door. I would roll my wheelchair to the bathroom door then climb out of the chair and crawl to the bathroom. Then I would lift myself onto the toilet.

My new disabled state limited my efforts outside of home to just going to the dialysis clinic every Monday, Wednesday, and Friday, but my girlfriend was extremely helpful in getting me out of the house to experience life with a disability. She explained to me that cities are obligated to accommodate people with disabilities in many ways, according to the Americans with Disabilities Act of 1990. I didn't realize before that ramps on sidewalks were there to provide wheelchair access. Before my amputations, I noticed these things, but I never had the need or the understanding to appreciate them. At first, I was embarrassed to go out in public in my wheelchair with no legs. Most children are astounded and stare, as if they or hypnotized; while most adults try to ignore the obvious elephant in the room.

Eventually, I grew accustom to people staring, and I would try to put myself in their position. I would ask myself, *What would I do if I saw someone with no legs?* It's not exactly something you would see every day, in the general population. After considering how others may view me, I had a bit more empathy for their position.

Climbing the stairs in Carlotta's house, where all the bedrooms were, wasn't an option for me, so I slept on a pull-out sofa in the living room. I never put the bed back in its sofa position, but I would make it every morning when I got up. It was hard making the bed, rolling around in my wheelchair, but I had to learn how to do these things, so I managed. Eventually, a physical therapist started to come every Tuesday and Thursday to teach me some exercises I could do to increase my strength. She told me it would be extremely important to build up my upper body strength in an effort to walk with prosthesis. I had many goals after my amputations of becoming independent, but my main goal was to walk again. Many things came with that goal, such as running, playing basketball, and riding a bike.

The next few months of my life were spent working out in a variety of ways, while waiting for my amputations to heal. Most of my workouts consisted of sitting in my wheelchair and using dumbbells. Then I would climb out of my wheelchair, on to the floor and do sit ups, leg lifts, and stretching exercises. During the day, I would go over to Hallmark Baptist Church in my wheelchair and do laps around the church. On one occasion, while I was at the church, I met a young man named Brandon, who was tending the grounds at the church. Brandon would see me doing my laps around the church, and he would bring me water. Little did he know I was on fluid restriction due to renal failure. Soon after we met, Brandon invited me to church.

About six months after my leg amputations, I had healed enough to where I could start being fitted for my first prosthesis. It was an exciting time for me. A wheelchair is a useful tool for people who can't walk, but it always gave me a sense of inferiority by looking up at others who were standing. I would rather stand and be face-to-face with a person I'm talking to. My prosthetist made a cast of both of my legs, and he told me it would take about three weeks to make the finished sockets. After my sockets were completed, I went to the office to try them on and try to walk for the first time in the last ten months.

When I first tried on my prosthesis, it was another out-of-body experience, thinking back to what I use to be (a good athlete, running in races every week, and playing in basketball leagues) to where I am now (a double below-the-knee amputee, trying to learn to walk again). I pulled my wheelchair up to the parallel bars, so I could use them for support. When I stood up for the first time as an amputee, it felt so unnatural, and I knew it would take a considerable amount of work just to stand on my own, let alone walking and running. I tried to take a few steps while holding on to the parallel bars, and it was difficult to say the least. My prosthetist suggested I take the prosthesis home and practice with a walker for a while.

Each day, I would go outside to the end of the driveway at my sister's house. After a few days, I extended my walk to the end of the block. It still didn't feel very natural, but I was getting an understanding of how to use prosthesis, to the point where it didn't seem so foreign. I started to practice walking inside the house with a cane. Walking with a cane was difficult, but I could tell I was getting stronger. Soon, I was walking to the end of the block, using my cane. Eventually, I would start going out into the community. I would go to stores and to the mall using my cane. Within a month of putting on my prosthesis for the first time, I was walking without any assistance.

I started therapy soon after I got comfortable with walking. When I first went to therapy, I assumed it would be more of what I was doing at home with walking around the block and going to the mall. The therapist and I talked about some expectations I should consider. One thing we talked about was *not* if I would fall, but when I would fall. My first assignment was to lie on the ground then stand back up on my feet. The upper body strength I had developed over the past few months helped me with this skill, and I was able to accomplish it with relative ease. The rest of therapy wasn't quite as easy. We climbed stairs, ascended and descended very steep inclines, and I also did some work on the treadmill.

At the beginning of therapy, I was much stronger than the first time I put on my prosthesis, but by the end of therapy, I was almost twice as strong as when I started. Therapy allowed me to envision my goals of running and playing basketball more clearly. Soon after therapy, I started to run a bit in the neighborhood, while walking. I found the prospect of running in the prosthesis that I had a bit cumbersome because they were extremely heavy. I was able to run, but not for a very long distance. I assumed that my work ethic displayed in my early days of athletics would benefit me in my quest to become a better runner.

My prosthetist suggested I attend an upcoming running clinic for amputees sponsored by Challenged Athletes Foundation. When I went to the clinic, I was amazed by all the people I had met who were living their lives as amputees. There were many children there whose condition was congenital, and it helped me realize how people can function at a high level, regardless of their condition. During the clinic, we learned several exercises used for runners with disabilities, and we had opportunities to compete with each other in several obstacle courses. At one point during an obstacle course, I was sweating so much that one of my prosthesis literally slipped off my stump. My sister, Carlotta, was with me at the clinic, and she was quite concerned about my ability to do things like run after she saw my leg come off while running.

While at the clinic, I spoke with some of the representatives from Challenged Athletes Foundation who suggested I apply for a grant to get some running prosthetics. Many people are familiar with this type of prosthesis, when during the 2012 Summer Olympics, a gentleman by the name of Oscar Pistorius competed in the 400 meters using these. I admit when I saw these prosthesis for the first time, I was somewhat intimidated by their appearance. I couldn't imagine how you could stand up in these things. I did apply for the grant, and soon after, I was approved and was able to receive my running legs.

Running with my regular prosthesis was a bit cumbersome to say the least, but I was able to manage while playing basketball and jogging. When I got the running legs, the difference was amazing. My prosthetist and I went to a high school track to see how they would feel. Putting the legs on initially was an experience in itself. Because the bottom of these prosthesis is round and not flat, keeping your balance is somewhat like balancing on ice skates for a novice skater. Eventually, I got the balance routine down, and I was able to stand in the prosthesis with no problems. I did learn you can't just stand still while wearing these type of prosthesis. Because of the round bottom, they literally force you to move almost to the point of running.

After I received my running legs, I began to run almost every day. Soon, I was running three to four miles, about four times a week. The running prosthesis were much lighter than my regular prosthesis, and they were more flexible. The difference in running between the two was like night and day. Before becoming an amputee, I spent most of my life as a runner, and I took for granted what running feels like. After I got the running legs, I was able to appreciate some of the small things that come with running—things like feeling the force of the wind against my face or just having the ability to move at a faster pace than walking. Even with my newly acquired disability, I felt somewhat empowered. Also, while I'm running, my mind-set is on a totally different level than my relaxed state of mind. Problem solving becomes clearer, the cares of this world seem to dissipate, and the issues I deal with every day seem to disappear. Sometimes when I'm running, I may forget that I'm an amputee or am suffering from renal failure.

My life was in a very good place. I didn't own a car, so I wasn't driving, but I used a city transportation service that catered to the disabled. So getting around town wasn't an issue. When I first started walking with my prosthesis walking was a chore, but by this time, it had become second nature for me. When I wore long pants while walking around town, most people couldn't tell I was an amputee, which was my goal from the beginning of this journey. The relationship with my girlfriend was going great, except we didn't see each other very often since she lived in Ohio, while I was in Texas. Our plan was to eventually get married and for me to move to Ohio because of her job.

RISE UP

I made the decision to go back to school and earn my bachelor's degree. My girlfriend was extremely supportive of the idea of getting my degree, but our relationship didn't hinge on my education. She accepted me for who I was in the place I was in. She had her master's degree, but she never made me feel inferior. Getting my degree was always something I wanted to do, and I felt I was capable of accomplishing. I began to look at several different avenues for achieving my goal of earning a degree. My first step was to visit the local community college in my area and speak to a counselor to advise me on what I should do. Since I had an associate's degree, the counselor suggested I concentrate my efforts on a four-year institution. Making a decision on school was determined by my lack of transportation, my current living situation, and the fact that I was planning to move to Ohio soon.

I made the decision that I would be going to school online, so I wouldn't have to worry about transportation to and from class. My next step was to find a school that would meet my needs. I wanted to find a program that would accept my past college credits, that was accredited and wouldn't take forever to get my degree. I looked at several programs until I found the Bachelors of Technical and Applied Studies at Ohio University. This program seemed to be perfectly suited to my needs. My plan was to move to northern Ohio. The school is in the southeastern portion of the state, so it would be more convenient for me. I also believed if I took two classes a semester, I could earn this degree in two to three years.

At the beginning of the summer of 2011, I was preparing myself to go back to school. I hadn't been to school in almost twenty years, so starting over again was a culture shock. Also, during that summer,

I began to do some work for a friend of mine. My friend had a contract with a prominent church in our area to design some flooring in the lobby and two entryways. This was in my line of expertise, so my friend reached out to me for help. My summer consisted of school preparation, working with my friend, and spending time with my girlfriend.

We didn't see each other very often, but she and I spoke on the phone on a daily basis. We made plans of eventually being together and getting married. We were attracted to each other physically, but we were also connected in heart and mind. For the first time in my life, I felt I was with my soulmate. Things were wonderful between us, until one day, in the summer of 2011, she went into the hospital for stomach pain. I've spent many days in the hospital, and it became routine. So when she was admitted, I didn't think much of it. A couple of days later, it was my birthday, and my girlfriend and I didn't speak on the phone. It was strange because we spoke on the phone every day up until that day. I was quite concerned, but I thought it had to be some reasonable explanation. The next day, my worst fears were realized when her sister called me to tell me she had passed away.

I was in complete and utter shock upon hearing this news. My life was finally in order, and we had planned to build our lives together. But it all just vanished into thin air. For days, it felt as if I was in a dream. I couldn't grasp the reality of her death.

My life was going through peaks and valleys. I had lost my legs, and I was back on dialysis. It was a low point in my life, and I had no idea of what was to become of me. Eventually, I learned to walk, to run, and to drive again. Also, I was getting ready to go back to school, get married, and move to Ohio. You can say I was at the top of the mountain once again. When I get the news of my girlfriend's death, everything came tumbling back down into the valley.

The plan after my amputations was to stay with my sister temporarily, until I got married and moved to Ohio. Unfortunately, I didn't have a plan B to fall back on when my girlfriend passed away. I made plans to go to Ohio for the memorial service. I had never been to a memorial service for one of my contemporaries, let alone someone whom I shared the most intimate aspects of my life. When I got to the church, I only expected to see members of her family and a few friends of hers, but upon entering the church, it was amazing to see the level of love and respect she had garnered from her community. I knew she was a wonderful human being whom I loved dearly, but I gained a new respect of how well she was received in her town, in her family, and in her career. They even started a scholarship at the community college, where she worked, in her honor. I was truly fortunate to have her in my life, if only for a brief period.

I made it back to Texas and had to pick up the pieces of my life and decide what I was going to do next. My sister and her family weren't putting any immense pressure on me to move, so I, at least, had a place to stay for the foreseeable future. School was starting in the fall of 2011, and I was still helping my friend with a couple of design projects. Needless to say, I was quite busy. With everything going on in my life, it provided a diversion from the death of my girl.

I began to develop a routine when I returned to Texas after the memorial service. Most of my days consisted of running at a nearby park, doing some design work with my friend, and preparing for school. The most daunting of all these task was my attempt to go back to school, seeing that I hadn't been to school in the past twenty years. My main issue was getting financial assistance to pay for my schooling. When I was in high school, my mother took care of things like this. I learned a bit from watching her help get all eight of her children into college. Through that experience, it helped me to get my son financial aid for college. So I had some experience in dealing with the institutions of higher learning in regards to financial aid.

My first collegiate experience was mainly funded by a group called the Texas Rehabilitation Commission, along with my parents. The rehab commission was able to help me because I was a diabetic, and that was considered a disability for which they could provide benefits. Because of my situation of being on dialysis and a double below-the-knee amputee, I thought I could use their services once again. My research indicated the group had changed their name from the Texas Rehabilitation Commission to Texas Department of Assistance and Rehabilitation Services, or DARS. I was extremely grateful for their help in my education at Kilgore College, but my research this time around found the group very inefficient and ineffective and full of bureaucratic red tape. Needless to say, they were not able to help me with my continuing education.

Due to my limited income, I was able to procure funds for school through grants and student loans. I wasn't too thrilled about getting loans that I would eventually have to pay back, but it was the only means available to get my bachelor's degree. By the fall of 2011, I was enrolled and taking classes at Ohio University. To think with my new disabilities, I could be embarking on another accomplishment gave me such a feeling of pride.

A routine was developed between school, some minor programming work with my friend, running, and spending time at the theater. These things occupied my time for the most part, so I was never without something to do. I had completely neglected my disabilities and made no provisions for things that could happen because of my disabilities.

Due to my problems with circulation, there was no way for me to get a natural port for dialysis called a fistula, so I had a Permacath. A Permacath is a plastic tube that's installed in your chest through an artery and extends outside your chest to allow the nurse to attach to the tubing from the dialysis machine. The problem with the Permacath is the potential for infection, and most physicians don't recommend using it for an extended period of time.

Unfortunately, I would find myself in the hospital at the most inopportune times because of an infection, usually when I had some assignment that was due. Sometimes, while lying in hospital beds, I would wonder if I had the ability to achieve this new goal I had set for myself—earning a bachelor's degree. I would start to think of excuses to justify why I should quit. Then I realized that none of the excuses could surpass the reasons why I had to accomplish this task. I had a legacy to leave to my son and my grandchildren of hard work and perseverance. I also wanted to provide hope to others that may be going through a difficult situation and feel as if they won't be able to accomplish a goal. When I realized the impact my graduating could have on my family, and society as a whole, there was no question that I had to finish.

After about two and a half years, I was able to complete my bachelor's degree at Ohio University, and I was so proud of the new accomplishment. As I said before, I did all my course work online, so I had never visited the campus. My next plan was to go to the campus and march in the graduation ceremony. None of my family would be able to travel to Ohio for the ceremony, but my son, Sean Junior was able to travel with me. We made plans to go a few days earlier than the ceremony so we would have an opportunity to see the city of Athens, Ohio, and visit the campus.

I thought it would be a good idea for Sean Junior and I to take this trip together because he and I didn't quite have the same relationship after his mother and I divorced. He was newly married, but his wife was very understanding about letting him go with me. The graduation ceremony was on Saturday, May 3, 2014, so we caught a flight out of DFW airport on Thursday morning, before the ceremony. We had a short layover in Atlanta on the way to Columbus, Ohio.

Watching Sean Junior during the trip, it seemed as if he was just along for the ride. But in my mind, it felt like we were on another journey together, like the old days, as father and son, when he was a small boy playing little league football or baseball, and I would take him on long road trips to games. Those were magical times that will be a source of fond memories. To capture some of those feelings again brought tremendous elation to my heart.

We arrived in Columbus around noon on Thursday, May 1, and we got our rent-a-car. Traveling was a main part of my work experience before all my health struggles, but I had never been to Columbus, Ohio, in all my travels. Neither of us had any knowledge of the city, so we were on an epic adventure together. The first order of business was to check into our hotel on the southwest side of Columbus. The hotel was right on the freeway headed to Athens, which was about the most convenience we could ask for. We couldn't get a hotel in Athens because everything was booked due to graduation.

After checking in, we went to dinner. After dinner we drove to Athens, so I could pick up my cap and gown. Upon entering the city, we noticed the Hocking River running alongside the Ohio University campus. To me, it was such a lovely sight to know that I'm a part of this wonderful institution. I could feel the goose bumps running up my arm. Athens is definitely a college town, and you can tell because of all the students walking around town. Once we arrived, I felt like part of the mix.

We cruised around town for a bit to get our bearings, then Sean Junior and I separated. I walked over to the building to pick up my cap and gown as many other students were doing. All the other students seemed so young. I was a bit embarrassed at my age, compared to the other graduates, but it didn't take away from my elation of getting my bachelor's degree. As I walked around campus and watched the young people getting ready to face the big world, a sense of pride started to overwhelm me because of my participation in the education process.

Sean Junior and I got back together, and we hit all the shops in town to pick up some Bobcat (the university mascot) paraphernalia. We bought hats and shirts that sported the Ohio University logo. I even purchased a stuffed bobcat for my granddaughter. That day's visit to the campus made me feel as if I was a part of the campus.

Eventually, we left the campus to drive around town, so we could find the dialysis center, where I would receive my dialysis treatment the next day. It wasn't far from campus. In fact, it was in a very convenient location in proximity to the campus. After we found the dialysis center, we decided to make the drive back to Columbus, to the hotel. The distance between Athens and Columbus is about seventy miles, one way. We would have to make this trip every day while we were in Ohio.

The next morning, we got up and drove back to Athens, so I could dialyze. The center was quite small compared to the one I go to in Fort Worth, but the nurses and technicians were very nice and professional. The center also had heated seats and Wi-Fi on the televisions, unlike the center in Fort Worth. I took a mental note to complain to the director in Fort Worth, so we can get some of these awesome amenities. One of the nurses told me her husband was also graduating from Ohio University with me. It gave the two of us a common interest. My dialysis experience, just like the rest of the trip, was going quite well.

The rest of that day was spent touring the campus and doing more shopping for miscellaneous Ohio University paraphernalia. Sean Junior and I spent much of our time learning about the campus and its history. By the time we were ready to drive back to Columbus, we had become Athenians. We spent the remainder of the evening in Columbus, having dinner and preparing for the graduation ceremony the next day.

The graduation ceremony was at 9:30 a.m. that Saturday, and they wanted the graduates to be there an hour early to get organized for the march into the convocation center. Plus, we had the seventy-mile drive from Columbus to Athens, which made for an early morning for us. I had forgotten to pack a belt for my dress pants, so I had to find a store to get a belt. The weather that morning, like most of the trip, was cool compared to Texas in May, but the forecast for later that morning was pleasant.

Sean Junior dropped me off at the convocation center, where I met with all my fellow graduates, and he found a parking space. I'm not sure how many people were in the graduating class that day, but it seemed like an enormous amount of people. We were all outside the center, and as far as the eye could see, there was a sea of black caps and gowns.

While standing outside with the other graduates, I met many of them. Most of them came from all around the state of Ohio, and many of them received their degrees online, like me. It was amazing to learn about the diverse backgrounds of the students. Most of them were shocked to learn I was from Fort Worth, Texas. They probably wondered why I would seek a degree from Ohio University and why I would travel so far for this ceremony, but of course, they didn't know my full story.

The people directing us on how we would enter the center and where we would sit told me we would have to climb a four-step staircase to get on stage to receive our degree. My problem was the staircase didn't have a banister. As an amputee, I climb stairs well as long as I have a banister to hold on to. Otherwise, I struggle a bit.

Needless to say, my anxiety was at an all-time high, thinking about climbing those stairs. The possibility of a misstep was real. At nine-thirty, we began the long procession into the convocation center, where many friends and family, including my son, were waiting to see their loved ones graduate. During the long walk in, all I could think about were those four-stair steps to the stage.

We took our seats after entering the convocation center. A young lady who was a graduate in our class sang the school song. Then the president of the university gave a short but inspiring speech. There was a guest speaker, a businessman from the Athens area, who gave the commencement speech. After his speech, we began our journey to the stage. Another long walk.

Once I got to the stage area, there were several people in front of me, and I had to stand there and wait until they called my name. I had to gather my composure and concentrate on the task at hand. When they called my name, I took a deep breath and started climbing. I made it to stage level without an incident and took another deep breath. I shook hands with the chancellor, who passed me a fake degree. I received the real degree in the mail a couple of months later. I was so elated after reaching another milestone in my life. A graduation is such a glorious occasion for everyone involved. As we walked outside the center, I saw all the congratulatory hugs and kisses as many of the graduates were meeting their loved ones. Finally, I saw my son through the multitude.

I felt the pride he had for his dad on this new accomplishment as we embraced. The whole trip was such a tremendous opportunity for Sean Junior and I to reconnect as father and son. I could have gotten my degree without participating in the ceremony, but I thought it was necessary for our relationship to make this trip together. We headed back to Columbus after the ceremony for dinner and to prepare for our trip back to Fort Worth.

Our flight the next day was in the late afternoon, so we got up the next morning, checked out of the hotel, and went over to the campus of Ohio State University, there in Columbus. It was an honor for both of us to be on the Ohio State campus since we were so familiar with their athletic program. Until we started walking around, we didn't realize how enormous the campus was. We saw all the sights, went to all the stores, and purchased more Ohio State paraphernalia.

The trip represented a turning point in my journey as a human being. Receiving the degree was a great accomplishment, but reconnecting with my son was by far the greatest part of the trip.

EPILOGUE

Many people told me, "You are the same person as you were before your amputation." But I contend that I'm truly not the same person. I'm extremely more aware of the world around me. I have a greater sense of tolerance. I'm much more sensitive to the plight of others. I've grown in many ways. I was considered a good person for most of my life, but circumstances have made me a better person.

When I first became an amputee, I would do everything I could to hide that truth. I would go to sporting attire websites to find pants to shroud my prosthesis. It was an attempt to look more athletic, and many who know me would tell me they couldn't tell I was an amputee. When I heard things like that, it would boost my ego. I would even work at great lengths to conceal my disability. One day at church, a gentleman came up to me and said, "I can tell you're an amputee because of the way you walk." I was so offended by his comment I just wanted to run away.

I think the shame I felt as an amputee came from what I experienced in the beginning years of my amputations. When I would go out in public, while on my wheelchair, I could just feel the eyes piercing my body as people would stare. I'm sure, as a nonamputee, I would have given the same peculiar looks to an amputee if they came into my presence. Most people just don't know how to respond to something different from what they're used to.

I've since grown in that area also. You know how some people say they wear their gray hair as a badge of honor. Well, I've been saying that for years now with all my gray. Now I'm wearing my prosthesis as a badge of honor to show others it's not the end of the world. There was a time when I wouldn't be seen in public with shorts on, but now, I wear shorts with a great sense of pride over what I've overcome.

My life, like many others, has been filled with triumph, tragedy, love, lose, pain, and jubilation; but I'm reminded of the apostle Paul, when he wrote in Philippians 4:11 "I have learned to be content in all circumstances." I've had the opportunity to meet many people in my life. Some of whom have had a profound influence on who I've become. The transformation from that small unassuming kid at "twenty-five oh-five Lucas Drive" to the person I've become has been truly amazing.

There is an old saying that "God doesn't give a person more than he can handle." Well, it seems as if He gave me a lot to handle, and I've managed to handle it to this point in my life. Years ago, my focus was on money and stability. Those things don't make a person selfish. Those things go a long way in this world. In fact, they can give you a certain amount of respect, but where do they leave us when our time runs out on this earth?

My joy comes when I meet someone who has lost all hope, and once they have had an encounter with me, seeing me walk or run or ride my bike with my prosthetics or just seeing the smile on my face despite my disabilities because God has allowed me to live an incredible life. I can sense a change that comes over them. Maybe, they forget about their current situation and focus on me. Maybe they wonder, "How this person before me can go through so much yet be so encouraging?" Then maybe, they will consider a loving God, who despite anything we can go through, He can provide hope in a hopeless situation.

As the days pass and time rolls on, I will eventually have to confront my mortality. I meet people today who are so encouraged by my story. I had a professor at Ohio University who was so amazed by my ability to walk and run after my amputations she, in turn, started to walk to work. What about someone years from now, who might pick this book up at some half-price bookstore on a discount shelf, and who's having a difficult time coping with life? The possibility gives me chills!

REFERENCES

National Institute of Diabetes and Digestive and Kidney Diseases Health Information Center, 1(800)860-8747, https://www.niddk. nih.gov/health-information/health-statistics/kidney-disease.

ABOUT THE AUTHOR

Sean B. Rice born June 17, 1963, the eighth child of Edgar & Exeree Rice in Fort Worth, Texas, at Saint Joseph Hospital. He attended elementary school in Fort Worth, Texas, until his family moved to Jefferson, Texas to take care of his grandfather. Sean has a son, a daughter-in-law, and 3 grandchildren. Sean attended Jefferson Middle and Junior high school until the eight grade. He graduated from Jefferson High School in 1981. Sean went on to college and received an Associate Degree in Drafting and Design Technology from Kilgore College in Kilgore, Texas. He received a Bachelors Degree in Technical and Applied Studies from Ohio University in Athens, Ohio. Sean excelled in his career as a Controls Engineer. He was a winning athlete in his favorite sports of football, basketball and track. At a young age Sean developed Type 1 diabetes (also known as juvenile diabetes) and followed all the rules for a healthy life. In 2003 he had a medical diagnosis of kidney failure and he went on dialysis. He was immediately put on the transplant list because he was a candidate in good physical condition for a successful kidney/pancreas transplant. Sean got a kidney/pancreas transplant at Baylor Hospital on March 4, 2004. It was the second pancreas transplant performed at the hospital. Six years later, the Kidney transplant failed and he had to go back on dialysis. Thankfully the pancreas is working well. The diabetes took a terrible toll on his body and he lost a finger a thumb and both legs. The loss did not discourage him. He was determined to conquer this setback. Sean was fitted with his prosthetic legs along with his running prosthesis and has competed in many 5k runs. With love and kindness for his fellowman, Sean treats each day as if it were his last. The ideal format for Sean is the written word, which is why he writes to inspire others to triumph and overcome the struggles in life.

—Shelia High

Received on 7/23/21 (but Had some online the same day I purch. it)
Finished reading 7/26/21

Wow, Abba!! :)

CPSIA information can be obtained
at www.ICGtesting.com
Printed in the USA
BVHW091355070521
606668BV00008B/1093

9 781644 684917